THE
COMPLETE
GUIDE TO
PSYCHIATRIC
DRUGS

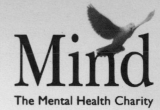

Mind
The Mental Health Charity

THE
COMPLETE
GUIDE TO
PSYCHIATRIC
DRUGS

A layman's guide to
anti-depressants, tranquillisers
and other prescription drugs

RON LACEY

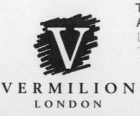

VERMILION
LONDON

First published in 1991 by Ebury Press
1 3 5 7 9 10 8 6 4 2

Copyright © Ron Lacey 1988, 1996

Ron Lacey has asserted his moral right to be identified as
the author of this work in accordance with the Copyright, Design and Patents Act, 1988

This revised edition published in
the United Kingdom in 1996 by Vermilion,
an imprint of Ebury Press, Random House,
20 Vauxhall Bridge Road, London SW1V 2SA

Random House Australia (Pty) Limited
20 Alfred Street, Milsons Point, Sydney
New South Wales 2061, Australia

Random House New Zealand Limited
18 Poland Road, Glenfield
Auckland 10, New Zealand

Random House South Africa (Pty) Limited
PO Box 2263, Rosebank 2121, South Africa

Random House UK Limited Reg. No. 954009

ISBN: 0 09 181367 0

Editor: Nicky Thompson
Design/make-up from disk by Roger Walker

Printed and bound in Great Britain
by Mackays of Chatham plc, Kent

Papers used by Vermilion are natural, recyclable products
made from wood grown in sustainable forests.

DEDICATION

This book is dedicated to two of my heroes. My father, Lance Bombardier Ron 'Badge' Lacey Rtd. was a war hero who, like Spike Milligan, did not speed victory in World War Two but probably delayed it for several seconds. Dad shared with Milligan the rare gift of being able to rejoice in the ridiculous. My other hero is the late Professor Derek Russell Davis. Derek was a long serving member of MIND's Council of Management whose influence and care was more often felt than seen. Derek was a gentleman and scholar in the truest sense.

Contents

Introduction

Approximately one quarter of all prescriptions dispensed by the National Health Service are for drugs which work on the central nervous system to alter our moods, states of mind and behaviour. The introduction of modern psychopharmaceuticals during the past 40 years has transformed and shaped our mental health services. Drugs are now central to the treatment of the variety of psychological states and conditions which are referred to collectively as mental illnesses or distress. When we go mad or feel desperately depressed the chances are that the first and often the only form of help offered to us will be a prescription for one of the drugs in this book. The purpose this guide is to inform the discussions that people have with their doctors, families, carers and advisers about their needs and choices. It should not be read as advice as to whether or how to use psychiatric drugs.

As well as describing the drugs this guide discusses the often unsatisfactory manner in which they are prescribed. This should not be read as an attack on the use of psychiatric drugs as such, or on psychiatry. It is an attempt to redress the balance of a dialogue about drugs which has been distorted by the uninformed prejudice and orchestrated panic about the needs of 'the mentally ill.' Psychiatric drugs are effective for most people for most of the time but they offer only symptomatic relief. High levels of social and emotional stress on vulnerable individuals and families can effectively undermine any benefits that these important and useful drugs can give.

Modern drugs have played a major part in improving the quality of our lives. The pharmaceutical industry makes a major contribution to the health and well being of the nation. We are fortunate to enjoy the benefits of a generally well regulated and dedicated medical profession. But there is no such thing as a perfect drug and there are as many saints, sinners and incompetents in the pharmaceutical industry and medical profession as in the rest of society. These days most of us know that all medicines have their side effects. Despite the gloom expressed by some about the state of modern society, there are signs that in some respects we are getting wiser with time and experience. It's not that long ago that we were happy to leave decisions about our health to the experts. If we got ill we took ourselves to the surgery and expected to get better simply by following doctor's orders. If we didn't get better we would put it down to bad luck. Nowadays we take a much more active role in looking after our health. This growing sense of personal responsibility is changing the expectations we have of our doctors. We now expect them to discuss the pros and cons of treatments with us rather than to give us instructions or orders. Many doctors welcome this change but others do not.

Our doctors have a common law duty to inform us about any proposed treatment in order to obtain our informed consent. But the law allows the doctor to exercise a degree of clinical judgement in deciding how much information he gives. This guide is based on the premise that we not only have rights to be sufficiently informed to give a valid consent to treatment but also we have a responsibility to ourselves to be as fully informed as possible. Both the law and common sense allow for exceptions to the principle of informed consent. An unconscious person or someone who is mad may be treated without their consent. In psychiatric medicine particular legal and social factors apply which distinguish it from all other branches of medicine. In writing this guide I have taken these factors into account. Put simply, because of the stigma which is attached to it, any diagnosis which falls within the broad remit of psychiatry is likely to put the sufferer at a serious disadvantage in many negotiations or interactions with others.

In certain circumstances a diagnosis of mental illness results in the patient losing the most basic of human rights – the right to liberty itself. Such a diagnosis also results in a person losing many of the rights of citizenship which most of us take for granted. To become a psychiatric patient means being subject to the power and often to the whims of those charged and empowered to provide care and treatment. Even without the formal trappings of disempowerment which ensues from a psychiatric diagnosis when we are labelled as 'schizophrenics', 'neurotics', 'depressives' or whatever, we are socially invalidated. If we complain about things we are as likely as not to be called 'paranoid'. We are often portrayed in the media as being helpless, hopeless or dangerous. If we stop taking our medication it is automatically assumed that we are too confused to appreciate its benefits.

This guide is strongly influenced by my work at MIND with and for people with mental health problems. When I joined the Association in 1975 most of the old asylums were still open but in a process of steady decay. Looking back now over two decades some things have changed for the better but some problems seem to be perennial. Many of the worst old institutions have closed. I believe that the grosser types of neglect and cruelty that were still all too common in them when I started at MIND are now very rare. However, we continue to be plagued with the same old public fear and prejudices about mental illness which fuelled the excesses of the old institutions and rendered their victims invisible non citizens. These old prejudices seem to have found new life in the moral panic which has ensued from inadequacies in community mental health services. Simplistic slogans about the 'needs of the mentally ill' are now used by shrill new voices of old institutional authoritarianism to challenge the small gains made by MIND and others toward promoting and protecting our civil and human rights when we become psychiatric patients. Informed consent is the key human rights issue which underlies this guide.

Cases like those of Christopher Clunis and Andrew Robinson, both of whom in psychotic states of mind killed innocent bystanders, understandably create public anxiety. However, these tragedies have been used to support a case for forcible drugging. No sensible person would argue that it would be wrong or unjust to detain a mentally ill person who presents a serious risk to self or others. Likewise, it would be naïve to rule out completely the prospect of administering an effective treatment to an individual who may lack insight and be dangerously mentally ill, if necessary without that person's consent. However, if powerful and potentially dangerous drugs are to be forced on a protesting patient, there are compelling moral obligations for all involved to be as certain as possible that the drugs are effective. Andrew Robinson killed whilst on a course of antipsychotic drugs as an inmate in a psychiatric unit.

Only a tiny minority of us are dangerous when we become mentally ill. More people are killed and injured by young men driving company cars under the influence of drink in a month than are killed and injured by the mentally ill in a decade. Most people who take psychiatric drugs are under no legal obligation to do so. Only a small (but growing) minority of patients in mental hospitals are subject to being compulsorily detained and may be thus liable to being lawfully treated without their consent. For the most part, consent is assumed rather than sought by prescribers and there are often powerful informal pressures on people to take their medicines. Such pressures may be exerted by nurses and other professionals or by relatives and carers. Pressures may take different forms from gentle encouragement to outright bullying. Some people whose accommodation is provided by local authorities or charities may have a condition incorporated into their licensing agreements to the effect that they must take their prescribed medications. The legality of such agreements in the context of the law of consent is questionable and the ethical considerations troublesome.

The use of informal pressures to encourage a person to take drugs prescribed for him may not always be wrong. Such gentle pressures may be totally justifiable in the context of a caring relationship with a vulnerable individual. But such pressures are not always be so benign either in intention or in their consequences for the person on the receiving end of psychiatric treatment. The quality of prescribing practices in psychiatry appears from published research evidence to be no less patchy than the quality of care in the community. Shortly after the first edition of this guide was published I was a co-author of a study[1] into people's experiences and views of receiving psychiatric services. This study took the form of in-depth interviews with 516 people who had each received at least one period of in-patient psychiatric treatment. The results of these interviews were then collated and compared with published research into the issues raised through our survey. We looked in detail at people's experience of being prescribed and taking psychiatric drugs.

Our findings confirmed many of our worst fears and experiences about the realities of being at the receiving end of psychia-

[1] Anne Rogers, David Pilgrim and Ron Lacey. *Experiencing Psychiatry – Users' Views of Services*. (Macmillan Press) 1993.

try. Prescribing practices which appeared to have as much in common with battery-farming techniques as individualised treatment programmes seemed to be the order of the day. We concluded that regardless of diagnosis 'Most patients appear to have received most of the available treatments (in particular drugs) for most of the time. Thus, whether diagnosed as suffering from schizophrenia or from depression, a majority (56.4 per cent) reported receiving antipsychotic medication, antidepressants and minor tranquillisers concurrently.' The concurrent use of antipsychotics with antidepressants is regarded by some respected authorities as controversial. They say that such drug cocktails may be of limited value therapeutically and they are likely to enhance the adverse effects of the individual drugs. In general the consensus among academic psychiatrists and psychopharmacologists seems to be that psychiatric prescriptions should be kept as simple as possible.

People prescribed psychiatric drugs are 'poor compliers'. That is to say that many people prescribed these drugs simply stop taking them. Fewer than half the prescriptions for antidepressants that are prescribed are actually taken. They are either thrown away or become dangerous hoards in medicine cabinets. In the case of antidepressants, particularly the older tricyclics and MAOIs, it is generally recognised that this is a consequence of their severe side effects in the early stages of treatment and the fact that it may take up to a month for them to exert their useful effects on depression. Some prescribers attribute poor compliance amongst their patients to their mental illness. They argue that such patients lack the insight to appreciate the benefits that their drugs bring to them and so stop taking them. Such judgements may be entirely sound but may not take account of the circumstances in which the drugs were prescribed. How often are patients' informed about the drugs being prescribed? Are they warned about side effects? Are prescribers sensitive to their patients' worries about side effects? People contacting MIND about drugs frequently complain about the lack of information about drugs they receive from prescribers and about their doctors' lack of interest or sympathy if they complain about side effects that they are experiencing.

When doctors take their own medicines

Psychiatrists obviously are aware of the side effects of the drugs they prescribe, but few seem able to describe from a subjective point of view what it actually feels like to take the drugs they prescribe for others. The literature is sparse but the following gems are worthy of retelling.

Haloperidol in Normals[2] is the tantalising title given to a paper published by two psychiatrists describing their personal experiences of haloperidol, a commonly prescribed antipsychotic drug used to treat conditions like schizophrenia. They injected one another with 5 milligrams of the drug, which is an average to low daily dose routinely given to patients. Haloperidol is one of the group of drugs which is commonly referred to as major tranquillisers. Normals in this context is the term used to denote that the subjects and authors of this study had not been diagnosed as suffering from any mental abnormality. The following account of the effects that these drugs had on the researchers illustrates why so many people reject the very idea that the term tranquilliser should be used as a classification for these powerful drugs. The two doctors reported that they experienced 'a marked slowness in thinking and movement' as well as 'profound feelings of inner restlessness'. Each reported a 'loss of will and a lack of physical and psychic energy'. Neither felt able to 'read, use the telephone or perform household tasks' of their own volition but they could perform them if instructed to do so. Neither experienced sleepiness or sedation; on the contrary both complained of 'severe anxiety'. Both felt incapable of doing their jobs for thirty-six hours. Whilst admiring the good doctors' spirit of enquiry I feel bound to note that the effects described by these 'normals' are identical to those so frequently complained of by people treated with haloperidol and other so called major tranquillisers.

View from the bottom[3] is the even more tantalising title of an article written by a psychiatrist describing his own experience of

---

[2] Belmaker, R.H. and Wald D.: 'Haloperidol in Normals,' *British Journal of Psychiatry*, 131, p.222, 1977.
[3] Anon, 'View from the bottom,' *Psychiatric Bulletin*, 14, p.452, 1990.

receiving treatment for severe depression as an in-patient in a psychiatric hospital. Resisting more mischievous explanations which suggest themselves for the author's choice of title, I assume that he used it to describe his perception of the nature of the relationship between the psychiatrist and the patient. As a psychiatrist he saw himself to be at the top of the hospital pecking order, whilst as patient he saw himself to be at the bottom. The thrust of the article was an appeal to his professional peers to be more sensitive to the subjective experiences of their patients. He writes of the side effects of antidepressants: 'It may be that the doctor can offer only symptomatic relief or none at all, but sympathetic enquiry itself can help the patient by legitimising his complaints. It is easy for a depressed patient to become preoccupied with problems such as thirst, tremor and clumsiness, constipation or urinary retention, which may be bad enough to cloud the picture of an improving mental state. The staff should also bear in mind the effect that the treatment, as well as the illness, may have on cognitive function, as this may be an added distress for a patient who cannot appreciate what is happening or the fact the impairment is temporary'.

I ate my mail was the headline in an American magazine which appeared in the early 70s in which a doctor described how he fed his addiction to tranquillisers by swallowing the copious quantities of free samples sent to him in the post by drug companies. This article appeared some ten years before the addictive potential of benzodiazepine drugs like Valium was acknowledged. The addictive properties of the benzodiazepines were brought to public attention by drug addiction treatment agencies, organisations concerned with alcohol abuse and by frustrated patients whose concerns had been dismissed by doctors for years.

Using this guide

This guide alone will **not** provide you with sufficient information to make the best decision for you in your circumstances as to whether or how you should use a psychiatric drug.

You should use the information in this guide to inform your discussions with your doctor or psychiatrist. Remember all drugs have side effects. Your discussions should focus on the questions on the next page.

1. What are the benefits of the drug?
2. What are its adverse effects?
3. How serious are these adverse effects?
4. Do the benefits of the drug substantially outweigh its adverse effects or any long-term hazards associated with its use?
5. How long should I expect it to take before I begin to feel the benefits of the drug?
6. Does the distress caused by the condition being treated outweigh the adverse effects of the drug and any long-term hazards it may have for me?
7. Are there any medicines, foods, or drinks I should avoid whilst taking the drug?
8. Are there any realistic alternatives to the drug?
9. How and when do I take the drug?
10. How and in what circumstances will I get the most benefit from the drug?
11. Who should I contact if I have any problems or worries about the drug?
12. How long should I expect to take the drug?
13. When should I next see the doctor to review my progress and my treatment?

PART ONE

Minor Tranquillisers

Introduction

Minor tranquillisers are prescribed to relieve anxiety and insomnia, as muscle relaxants and for the treatment of epileptic fits. They are also used by dentists to calm nervous patients. The most commonly prescribed minor tranquillisers are a group of products called the benzodiazepines. The two best known of these are Valium and Mogadon. There are very few real differences between benzodiazepine products and all have similar effects. As well as the benzodiazepines there are a number other compounds which are prescribed for anxiety and sleep problems but these are much less often prescribed.

Minor tranquillisers were massively over-prescribed for two decades and many thousands of people have become hooked on them. According to a MORI poll published in 1985[1] by the BBC 23 per cent of Britain's adult population has taken a minor tranquilliser at least once. Of those, 35 per cent, or approximately 3.5 million people, had taken them for periods of four months or longer. Four months is long enough for people to become hooked on these drugs and it is doubtful whether they have any useful effects as tranquillisers after this period. Not everyone who takes these drugs gets hooked on them. Some research suggests that approximately half of long-term tranquilliser users will have difficulty in withdrawing from them; others put the numbers one in three and others at one in eight. Applying these estimates to the MORI poll figure of 3.5 million long-term

[1] Lacey, R. and Woodward, S.: *That's Life! Survey of Tranquillisers.* BBC Publications, London, 1985.

benzodiazepine users gives us a figure of between 435,000 and 1.75 million people who may have become hooked.

The story of the minor tranquillisers illustrates the dangers inherent in seeking simple medical solutions to complex social and emotional problems. Before the advent of the benzodiazepines, other frequently lethal drugs were being overprescribed and overused. These were the barbiturates which had over a period of time been discovered to be highly addictive and to have a potentially fatal withdrawal syndrome. The barbiturates can be lethal in overdose and many people, particularly elderly people, were becoming dangerously confused and dying as the result of unintentionally and unknowingly taking overdoses of barbiturate compounds. Eventually a pressure group called CURB was set up by doctors which campaigned for a substantial reduction of the use of the barbiturate compounds. The scandal of the barbiturates and the continuing demand for happy pills created an ideal climate in which a new 'safe', 'non addictive' minor tranquilliser with 'few adverse effects' could be launched. That drug was chlordiazepoxide, better known by its trade name of Librium, the first of the benzodiazepine tranquillisers, and introduced in 1960.

Librium was discovered accidentally by a chemist called Sternbach who in the course of clearing out a laboratory came across a number of compounds for which no use had then been found. Amongst these was chlordiazepoxide, which he sent for pharmacological tests to see whether it might have some useful pharmaceutical properties. This 'happy accident' led to the biggest money-making bonanza in the history of medicine. Chlordiazepoxide was found to have useful sedative, muscle-relaxant and anticonvulsant properties. One researcher noted that 'A taming effect was observed in rhesus monkeys, which can be very vicious in captivity'. A new safe and 'cure-all' was launched on to a sellers' market left by the discrediting of the barbiturates. A now notorious advertisement for chlordiazepoxide proclaimed 'Whatever the diagnosis...Librium'. Another advertisement for one of Librium's many chemical cousins bore a picture of a depressed housewife seated behind mops, brooms and other household tools set out like symbolic prison bars. The caption to this advertisement read 'You can't set her free, but you can help her feel less anxious'. The story of the marketing of the benzodiazepines is told by Charles Medawar, a leading critic and commentator of the pharmaceutical industry in his book *Power and Dependence*.[2]

Benzodiazepine products were promoted as solutions to just about every problem known to man and woman (with the emphasis on woman!). Tensions between grandparents and grandchildren could now be cured by the pills. A young woman leaving home and going to university was also a situation in which a doctor might helpfully intervene with a prescription. 'A whole new world of anxiety ... Her newly awakened intellectual curiosity may make her more anxious about international and domestic events'. Such advertising to doctors might be thought laughable had it not been so successful in terms of hundreds of millions of prescriptions they wrote worldwide. Millions of pills were distributed free to doctors and to teaching hospitals in order to establish brand names. All this added up to one of the most successful and profitable marketing exercises ever. It is a sobering thought that market forces might be as influential in determining nature of our health services as our health needs. Inappropriately prescribed tranquillisers not only caused a major addiction problem; they also incurred a terrible waste of health service money. The only parties who profited from this sorry saga were the shareholders of the drug companies concerned.

Minor tranquillisers can be very useful drugs and are relatively safe when taken on their own. Their side effects are usually less severe than those of other prescribed mood-altering drugs. But they have been and still are overused and overprescribed, and their problems and hazards considerably outweigh their benefits. Minor tranquillisers are most commonly prescribed as sleeping tablets. They are often taken for years on end despite the fact that they cease to be effective after about two weeks. After this period many people find that if they try to stop taking them their insomnia is even worse than when they began taking the pills. Insomnia is major withdrawal effect of sleeping pills. Thus, people can be trapped in a vicious spiral of pill-taking. As a result they will be less alert, their memories will be less reliable, they will be more accident prone and may experience sudden explosions of rage or violent behaviour.

---

[2] Medawar, Charles. Power and Dependence Social Audit on the safety of medicines. Social Audit Ltd. 1992.

The use of pills to deal with insomnia more often than not obscures its causes. Insomnia is a symptom not a disease. Inadequate exercise, too much coffee, inappropriate sleep patterns, unresolved worries, boredom, grief and pain can all cause sleep disturbances but none of these can be resolved by pills. Elderly people in particular are likely to be prescribed sleeping pills. After retirement people's life rhythms are disrupted. They get less exercise, the routines they adapted to during their working lives come to an end, they may have catnaps during the day or fall asleep in front of the television, so that when they go to bed they are unable to sleep. Lying awake when the rest of the world is asleep becomes a problem, anxieties tend to mount and make things progressively worse. There are very effective non drug-based solutions to insomnia which involve teaching people to manage their sleep. However, the domination of the prescription pad in health care means that they are less well known and available than they should be.

Minor tranquillisers are prescribed three times more frequently to women than to men. Some believe this to be a consequence of a male-dominated medical profession which sees women as being more emotional or more neurotic than men. Others argue that women's lives are inherently more stressful than those of men. The view that women should be constitutionally more prone to emotional disorders than men does not on the surface seem very logical. Such a view is not borne out by any body of systematic research. In this area there appear to be more questions than answers. Why are single women less prone to depression than married women? This pattern is reversed for men. Married men are less prone to depression than single men. Why should marriage be bad for women's mental health and good for men's? Many women's work consists of caring for their families and homes. Caring for children and dependent relatives may be infinitely more stressful than a man's work. Men may complain about their jobs but those jobs do offer them clear and valued roles as well as a variety of experience and human contact. Being a carer is usually a very isolated role. Caring for a demanding child or an elderly relative is all the more stressful because it involves love and a degree of personal commitment far in excess of anything required by paid employment. Traditional 'women's work' is not governed by a 35-hour week, or by conditions set down by any health and safety regulations. In the light of such realities the tranquilliser advertisement which proclaimed 'You can't set her free but you can help her feel less anxious' has a decidedly uncomfortable ring to it!

Benzodiazepine minor tranquillisers are marketed as either 'hypnotics' or 'anxiolytics', but there is little or no difference between them other than the length of their half-lives i.e., the time it takes for the body to excrete half the active drug). A short-acting drug is active, therefore, for a shorter period of time than a long-acting one. In some circumstances a short-acting tranquilliser may be preferable to a long-acting one because it is less likely to cause a hangover the following day. Such differences may make one benzodiazepine more useful than another, but the real differences between the differently labelled pills are as subtle as the difference between a brick and a half brick. Most benzodiazepines are metabolised by our bodies into the same active substances. In the following list of benzodiazepine tranquillisers, the different products are divided into hypnotics and anxiolytics, and then further divided into long- and short-acting compounds. The side and withdrawal effects are listed for the group as a whole.

Getting the most from minor tranquillisers

- If you have been taking tranquillisers for more than two months, don't suddenly stop taking them – do it gradually, and preferably with the help of your doctor.
- Use sleeping pills for as short a time as possible and remember that after between three and fourteen days your body has adjusted to them and they will no longer be helping you to sleep. If you are persistently unable to sleep you should consider whether your lifestyle and diet are causing your difficulties. If you must take sleeping pills, do so intermittently. You will be doing your brain no good at all by embarking on a career of pill-taking.
- Use anxiety-relieving pills for as short a time as possible and remember that they are more likely to have negative rather than positive effects on your life if you take them for too long. Ask yourself why you continue to feel anxious and whether you are really using the pills as a means to avoiding looking at what is really causing your anxiety. If you must take them, do so intermittently – use them as you would use an aspirin, that

is, when you really must relieve a pain, and until you can get the cause of the pain looked at.
- Don't believe anyone who tells you that your insomnia or anxiety are caused by a chemical imbalance in your brain.
- Minor tranquillisers should not be used to treat children except in very rare circumstances, such as night terrors.

Benzodiazepine Minor Tranquillisers

Long-acting benzodiazepines prescribed for sleep problems

FLUNITRAZEPAM

Trade name	Description	Dose
Rohypnol	1 mg purple tablets	0.5–1 mg per day.

FLURAZEPAM

Trade name	Description	Dose
Dalmane	15 mg grey/yellow capsules. 30 mg black/grey capsules.	15–30 mg per day.
Paxane	15 mg green/grey capsules. 30 mg green/black capsules.	

NITRAZEPAM

Trade name	Description	Dose
Mogadon	5 mg purple/black capsules.	5–10 mg per day
Somnite	Off-white liquid to be taken orally.	5–10 mg per day.
Surem	5 mg mauve/grey capsules.	5–10 mg per day.
Under generic name	5 mg white tablets. Liquid to be taken orally.	5–10 mg per day.

General information
Long-acting drugs may be more likely to cause hangovers and have less severe withdrawal effects. Elderly and physically frail people should use half the above doses. These drugs can impair reflexes and the ability to drive.

Short-acting benzodiazepines prescribed for sleep problems

LOPRAZOLAM

Trade name	Description	Dose
Under generic name	1 mg white tablets.	Initially 1 mg per day increased to 1.5–2 mg per day.

TEMAZEPAM

Trade name	Description	Dose
Under generic name	10 mg white tablets marked TMZ 10	10–20 mg at bedtime
	20 mg white tablets marked TMZ 20	Elderly or frail 10 mg at bedtime 20 mg in exceptional circumstances.
Temazepam elixir	Green lemon mint flavoured liquid containing 10 mg of temazepam per 5 ml.	

General information

Less likely than long-acting compounds to cause hangover but withdrawal effects may be more severe. Elderly and physically frail people should take half the above doses. These drugs can impair reflexes and the ability to drive.

Long-acting benzodiazepines prescribed for anxiety

ALPRAZOLAM

Trade name	Description	Dose
Xanax	250 microgram white tablets. 500 microgram pink tablets.	250–500 micrograms three times daily, increased if necessary to a total of 3 mg per day.

BROMEZAPAM

Trade name	Description	Dose
Lexotan	1.5 mg lilac tablets. 3 mg pink tablets.	3–18 mg per day in divided doses. (In rare cases up to 60 mg per day may be given to hospital in-patients.)

CHLORDIAZEPOXIDE

Trade name	Description	Dose
Librium	5 mg green/yellow capsules. 10 mg green black capsules. 5 mg greenish yellow tablets. 10 mg light bluish green tablets. 25 mg dark bluish green tablets.	10 mg three times per day increased if necessary to 60–100 mg per day
Under generic name	5 mg, 10 mg and 25 mg white tablets.	

CLORAZEPATE DIPOTASSIUM

Trade name	Description	Dose
Tranxene	7.5 mg maroon/grey capsules 15 mg pink/grey capsules.	7.5–22.5 mg per day in divided doses.

DIAZEPAM

Trade name	Description	Dose
Valium	2 mg white tablets. 5 mg yellow tablets. 10 mg blue tablets. Injections. Suppositories.	2 mg three times daily increased if necessary to 15–30 mg per day in divided doses. For children with night terrors 1–5 mg at bedtime.
Under generic name	2 mg and 5 mg white tablets. Liquid containing 2 mg per 5 ml. Liquid containing 5 mg per 5 ml.	

General information

Withdrawal effects with this group of drugs are less severe than those of the short-acting benzodiazepines. However they do have a potential for addiction and so they should be taken with care for periods of days rather than weeks. Elderly or physically frail people should receive half the adult dose. These drugs can impair the memory reflexes and the ability to drive.

Short-acting benzodiazepines prescribed for anxiety

LORAZEPAM

Trade name	Description	Dose
Ativan	1 mg blue tablets. 2 mg yellow tablets. Injection.	1–4 mg per day in divided doses.

OXAZEPAM

Trade name	Description	Dose
Under generic name	10 mg white tablets marked WY 013.	15–30 mg per day i divided doses. Elderly or frail people 10–20 mg per day.
	15 mg white tablets marked WY 013.	Not recommended for children.

General information

Short-acting compounds may have more severe withdrawal effects than long-acting ones. Withdrawal is best managed by switching to a long-acting compound for a planned gradual withdrawal. Elderly and physically frail people should use half the above doses. These drugs can impair reflexes, memory and the ability to drive.

Benzodiazepine minor tranquillisers: side effects and further information

Common side effects

Feelings of tiredness, drowsiness and an inability to concentrate. Impairment of memory. Difficulty in co-ordinating movements. Ataxia (shaky movements and unsteady gait caused by the brain's failure to control the body's posture and the strength and direction of limb movements). Confusion (more likely in elderly people). Excitement, restlessness and aggressive behaviour.

Withdrawal

Withdrawal effects are: Anxiety. Insomnia. Agitation. Palpitations. 'Jelly legs'. Aches and pains. Restlessness. Panic attacks.

Sweating. Tremors. Pins and needles. Loss of appetite. Tension. Occasionally, convulsions.

Conditions in which benzodiazepines should be used with caution

Respiratory disease. Muscle weakness. History of drug abuse. Pregnancy (particularly in the first three months). Breast-feeding. The elderly and physically frail should take reduced doses. Kidney and liver disease. Minor tranquillisers should not be taken over long periods of time.

Use in pregnancy and breast-feeding

There may be an increased risk of a baby being born with a cleft palate if the mother is taking a benzodiazepine during the first three months of her pregnancy. Children of mothers taking benzodiazepines may be born suffering from the 'floppy baby syndrome', a condition in which the child is withdrawn, drowsy, listless and seemingly indifferent to feeding. This condition improves once the drug has been excreted from the baby's system. If the mother has taken benzodiazepines throughout her pregnancy, there is the risk that a newly born child could be exposed to the withdrawal effects. The drugs also pass from mother to infant in the breast milk, which can cause weight loss and lethargy in the baby. The long-term effects of a mother's chronic use of benzodiazepines during pregnancy on her unborn child's development have not been fully monitored.

Elderly people and benzodiazepines

As we grow older our bodily functions slow down, which often means that any drugs we consume will remain in our bodies for longer. In some circumstances this may not be a problem, but in others it can cause serious complications. There have been a number of scandals in old people's homes involving the over drugging, whether by accident or design, of residents. The quality of prescribing in old people's homes in the recent past has been shown to leave much to be desired. As benzodiazepines may take much longer than normal to leave an elderly person's system, the regular use of tranquillisers can result in the amount of the drug being gradually built up to dangerous levels. When taking these drugs elderly people may also be much more prone to falls resulting in serious injuries. Concern about this type of accident has been voiced in the medical press by orthopaedic surgeons. Elderly people are more vulnerable to suffering from the side effects of drugs and great caution is required in the way that drugs are prescribed and administered. As well as benzodiazepines, there are several other minor tranquillisers which are prescribed for the treatment of anxiety and insomnia. Their properties and effects are listed below.

HOW BENZODIAZEPINES INTERACT WITH OTHER DRUGS AND MEDICINES

Drug	Interaction
Alcohol	Increased sedation and increased intoxication.
Anaesthetics	Increased sedation.
Opioid painkillers such as codeine, pethidine, morphine	Increased sedation.
Antidepressants. Anti-epileptic drugs. Antihistimines, for example common cold treatments, travel sickness pills, nasal inhalants, treatments for nettle rash	Increased sedation. Reduces effect of clonazepam. Increased sedation.
Drugs to reduce blood pressure	Increased reduction in blood pressure.
Antipsychotics	Increased sedation.
Disulfiram (a drug used to treat alcoholism)	Increased sedation with chlordiazepoxide and diazepam.
Levodopa (a drug used to treat Parkinsonism)	Benzodiazepines may reduce effectiveness of levodopa.
Cimetidine (a drug used to treat ulcers)	Increased level of benzodiazepines in the blood stream.

Other drugs prescribed for anxiety

BUSPIRONE

Trade name	Description
Buspar	5 mg white tablets (engraved with) 5.
	10 mg white tablets (engraved with) 10.

General information

Buspirone is a relatively new drug for the treatment of anxiety, having been in use in Britain since 1985. In these circumstances it may be some time before we know how valuable buspirone really is. It appears to have a number of advantages over the benzodiazepines, as well as a few disadvantages. It is said that buspirone does not cause sedation or physical dependence, impair physical skills or co-ordination, and that it is safe in overdose. The major disadvantage it appears to have is that it may take up to four weeks before it relieves anxiety. As it does not cause sedation, buspirone has no place in the treatment of insomnia. How the drug exerts its effects is unknown. Like all the drugs in this group, it can impair reflexes and the ability to drive.

Dosage information

Adult (16 and over): Treatment begins with 5 mg two to three times daily, which may be increased if necessary every two or three days to the usual dose range of between 15-40 mg per day. **The maximum dose is 45 mg per day.**
Elderly and physically frail: The maximum dose for elderly people is 30 mg per day.

Side effects and further information

The side effects of buspirone are said to become less severe with time. If side effects do become a problem, the manufacturers recommend a reduction in dose. According to the manufacturers, 'the only side effects that occurred with significantly greater frequency with buspirone treatment than with a placebo were dizziness, headaches, nervousness, lightheadedness, excitement and nausea. Tachycardia (increased heart rate), palpitations, chest pain, drowsiness, confusion, dry mouth, fatigue, sweating and clamminess have also been reported rarely'.

Conditions in which buspirone should be avoided
Epilepsy. Severe liver or kidney disease. Pregnancy and breast-feeding. It should not be used concurrently with MAOI (Monoamine oxidase inhibitor) antidepressants.

Conditions in which buspirone should be used with caution
When there is a history of liver or kidney disease. Buspirone is of no use in the treatment of the withdrawal effects of benzodiazepines.

CHLORMEZANONE

Trade name	Description
Trancopal	200 mg yellow tablets.

General information
Chlormezanone is a mildly sedating compound which may be used for the short-term treatment of anxiety, insomnia and muscle spasms. It may be prescribed with painkillers to relieve conditions like arthritis. It is a sedating drug that can cause drowsiness. When used for sleep disorders it may have a hang-over effect of drowsiness the following day. It can also impair reflexes and the ability to drive.

Dosage information
Adult (16 and over): 200 mg three to four times per day, or 400 mg in a single dose at bedtime.
Elderly and physically frail: Elderly people should take half the adult dose.
Children: Not recommended for children.

Side effects and further information
Drowsiness and lethargy. Dizziness. Nausea. Headache. Dry mouth. Rashes. Jaundice. If used for more than a few weeks dependency can occur.

Conditions in which chlormezanone should be avoided
Serious lung disorders. Depressed breathing. Porphyria (a rare blood disorder which causes severe sensitivity to sunlight, resulting in inflammation or blistering of the skin, inflammation of the nerves, severe mental disturbances, blue urine and attacks of stomach pain).

Conditions in which chlormezanone should be used with caution

Respiratory disease. Where there is a history of drug dependency. Muscular weakness. Pregnancy and breast-feeding (see below). The elderly and physically frail should receive reduced doses. It should only be used for short-term treatment and should be withdrawn gradually.

Use in pregnancy and breast-feeding

There are no reports of damage to the unborn child but if the mother takes this drug for long periods of time during pregnancy, the foetus will be exposed to sedation and the risk of dependence which could lead to the new-born baby experiencing withdrawal effects.

HYDROXYZINE

Trade name	Description
Atarax	10 mg orange tablets.
	25 mg green tablets.
	Syrup to be taken orally.

General information

Hydroxyzine is used for the short-term relief of anxiety and insomnia. It may also be used to enhance the effect of painkillers and in the treatment of asthma. Rather unusually for this group of drugs, hydroxyzine is said to have little potential for causing dependence. Like all the drugs in this group, however, it can impair reflexes and the ability to drive. Some patients may have a sensitive reaction to this drug.

Dosage information

Adult (16 and over): 50–100 mg per day.
Elderly and physically frail: The elderly and physically frail should receive a lower dose.
Children: Not recommended for children.

Side effects and further information

The side effects of hydroxyzine are said to be mild and infrequent. The most commonly reported side effects are disturbances of vision, drowsiness and itching.

Conditions in which hydroxyzine should be avoided
Sensitivity to hydroxyzine. Pregnancy (see below).

Conditions in which hydroxyzine should be used with caution
Caution should be exercised in using the drug concurrently with barbiturates, alcohol, opiates and other tranquillisers.

Use in pregnancy and breast-feeding
Avoid using in pregnancy, particularly during the first three months. Studies in animals have shown risks to the foetus but these have not been confirmed in humans. Nevertheless, as with all sedating drugs, there is a risk that the unborn and newly born may be adversely affected.

MEPROBAMATE

Trade name	Description
Equanil	200 mg white tablets.
	400 mg white tablets.

General information
Meprobamate is less effective than the benzodiazepines as a tranquilliser, it is more dangerous in overdose, more likely to cause dependence and has more severe withdrawal effects. Meprobamate may have some uses but it is difficult to see what these may be, given that there are many other less problematic compounds available within this group.

Dosage information
Adult (16 and over): 400 mg three to four times a day.
Elderly and physically frail: Elderly people should receive half the adult dose or less.
Children: Not recommended for children.

Side effects and further information
Meprobamate has a wide range of side effects and these are more frequent and more hazardous than those of the benzodiazepine group. It is also potentially addictive as tolerance develops rapidly, which means that increased doses may be required to achieve the drug's marginal benefits. If the drug is used over any length of time the patient may develop a craving for it. The with-

drawal effects of meprobromate are: Drowsiness. Light headedness. Confusion. Ataxia (shaky movements and unsteady gait
caused by the brain's failure to control the body's posture and the
strength and direction of limb movements). Impaired memory.
Headaches. Vertigo. Dry mouth. Stomach upsets. Reduced urination. Agranulocytosis (a serious deficiency of white blood cells
caused by damage to the bone marrow). Allergic reactions. Convulsions. Paradoxically, excitement. Paraesthesia (pins and needles). Tolerance to the effects of the drug leading to addiction.

Withdrawal

Not every patient experiences withdrawal effects, but many do.
The effects may be sufficiently severe to be life-threatening if left
untreated. The effects are: Anxiety. Feelings of weakness. Tension. Loss of appetite. Epileptic fits. Delirium. Hallucinations.
Sudden withdrawal may cause fits.

Conditions in which meprobromate should be avoided

Severe lung and breathing problems. Pregnancy and breast-
feeding. Porphyria (a rare blood disorder which causes severe
sensitivity to sunlight, resulting in inflammation or blistering of
the skin, inflammation of the nerves, severe mental disturbances
and attacks of stomach pain). Meprobamate should only be used
for severe problems when no alternative treatment is available.

Other drugs prescribed for sleep problems

CHLORAL HYDRATE

Trade name	Description
Noctec	500 mg clear orange-red capsules.
Chloral mixture	Foul-tasting liquid, to be diluted and taken orally.
Chloral elixir Paediatric	Foul-tasting liquid with blackcurrant flavour, to be diluted and taken orally.
Welldorm	Bluish-purple capsule containing 707 mg chloral betaine, which is the equivalent of 414 mg of chloral hydrate.
Welldorm elixir	Foul-tasting red liquid with passion-fruit flavour, to be diluted and taken orally.

General information

The use in psychiatry of chloral hydrate goes back to the last century; it is mentioned in a psychiatric textbook written in 1899 by Emil Kraepelin, one of the leading pioneers of modern psychiatry. His brief entry on the drug reads: 'Chloral hydrate: Induces longer sleep, sometimes with drowsiness in the morning. Mordant, unpleasant taste'. It does indeed have an extremely bitter and unpleasant taste which is barely concealed by the fruit flavours added to make it more palatable. If it comes into contact with the skin it can cause irritation.

Chloral hydrate is used in the short-term treatment of insomnia. The treatment of insomnia in children by drugs is controversial, but if it is necessary the treatment should not be given for longer than one or two days at a time. If the problem persists it is wise to seek non-medical methods of treatment. Behaviour therapy has been successfully used to treat sleeping difficulties in infants and children. Quite often insomnia in children can be traced to anxieties caused by difficulties being experienced by their parents. In such circumstances the use of drugs not only fails to address the underlying anxieties causing the insomnia, but unnecessarily exposes the child to the hazards of drugs. In comparison with other drugs used to treat insomnia, chloral hydrate is relatively safe, but in long-term use it can lead to dependence and addiction.

Dosage information

Adult (16 and over): Chloral mixture: 5–20 ml taken 15 to 30 minutes before bedtime.

Noctec: 500 mg–1 g. One to two capsules to be taken at bedtime with plenty of water.

Welldorm capsules: One to two capsules at bedtime.

Welldorm elixir: 15–45 ml taken 15 to 30 minutes before bedtime.

The maximum daily dose is 2 g with plenty of water.

Elderly and physically frail: Should receive same doses as for adults.

Children: Chloral mixture: For children aged one to five, 2.55 ml; aged six to twelve, 5–10 ml, taken 15 to 30 minutes before bedtime.

Chloral elixir (paediatric): For children up to one year old, 5 ml well diluted.

Noctec: Not recommended for children.

Welldorm capsules and elixir: Doses are calculated by body weight: 30–50 mg and 1–1.7 ml per kilogram of body weight.

Side effects and further information

Chloral hydrate quite commonly causes stomach upsets. Although rare, it can also cause rashes, headache, ketonuria (the presence of acetone in the urine), excitement and delirium. Long-term use may cause kidney damage and dependence. Avoid contact with skin. Avoid long-term use and abrupt withdrawal.

Conditions in which chloral hydrate must be avoided

Severe heart disease. Upset stomach. Serious liver or kidney disease.

Conditions in which chloral hydrate should be used with caution

Where there is a history of drug dependence. Pregnancy and breast-feeding (see below). Lung or respiratory disease.

Use in pregnancy and breast-feeding

Like other drugs chloral hydrate passes from the mother to the foetus in the womb and from the mother to the newly born child through breast milk. In the unlikely event that a mother takes chloral hydrate for prolonged periods during pregnancy the unborn child will be exposed to all of the effects listed above.

CHLORMETHIAZOLE

Trade name	Description
Heminevren	192 mg greyish brown capsules. Colourless syrup containing 50 mg chlormethiazole per 50 ml.

General information

Chlormethiazole is a short acting drug used for the short-term treatment of severe insomnia and agitation in the elderly where no other drug is available or effective. It is also used in the treatment of alcohol withdrawal. In general caution is urged in the use of this drug as it has a high potential for addiction. (Although it seems that amongst a good number of practitioners in the field of addiction the exchange of one addiction for another is quite acceptable!) The use of this drug may seriously impair driving the day after it has been taken.

Dosage information
Severe insomnia in the elderly: 1–2 capsules or 5–10 ml at bedtime. Severe agitation in the elderly: 1 capsule or 5 ml three times daily.
Not recommended for children.

Side effects and further information
Chlormethiazole can cause similar effects to a heavy cold ie., a runny nose and watering eyes. Other common side effects include: headache, upset stomach and dependence on the drug. Less often people may get very high and excited. Other reported side effects include: skin rashes, blisters and allergies. Not everyone experiences all of these effects.

Conditions in which chlormethiazole should be avoided
Severe chest or breathing problems. Alcoholics and people with serious drink problems should not be prescribed this drug. Should not be used to treat children.

Conditions in which chlormethiazole should be used with caution
Heart disease, liver disease and kidney disease. Caution should also be used if people are being treated with drugs which affect the central nervous system. Should only be used for short-term treatment.

Use in pregnancy and breast-feeding
Chlormethiazole should not be used during pregnancy or whilst breast-feeding.

TRICLOFOS

Trade name	Description
Triclofos elixir	Liquid to be taken 30 minutes before bedtime.

General information
Triclofos is a derivative of chloral hydrate and has similar effects, although it is less likely to cause stomach ulcers. For details of effects and side effects, see the entry for chloral hydrate.

Dosage information
Adult (16 and over): 1–2g 30 minutes before bedtime. The maximum daily dose is 2 g.

Elderly and physically frail: The elderly and physically frail should receive reduced doses.
Children: For children up to 1 year of age, 100–250 mg; between one and five years old, 250–500 mg; and between six and twelve years old, 500 mg-1 g.

ZOLPIDEM

Trade name	Description
Stilnoct	5 mg round glossy white tablets.

General information
Zolpidem is a recently introduced drug with similar but different effects to benzodiazepine sleeping pills. It acts faster than other similar drugs and so people are advised to take it immediately before sleep. It has a very short half and thus is a short-acting drug. For this reason it is less predictable than other drugs in terms of the length of sleep it induces. The drug's short period of action reduces the risk of morning-after residual effects. It is thought that zolpidem may not have the same potential for causing dependency but as with all sleeping pills caution is advised against using them for more than a few days at a time. Zolpidem may affect driving skills the morning after use and may enhance the effects of alcohol.

Dosage information
Adult: 10 mg at bedtime.
Elderly or physically frail: 5 mg
Children: Not recommended for children.

Side effects and further information
Nausea and upset stomach, dizziness, headache, depression, memory disturbances. Loss of energy, nightmares, confusion, trembling and clumsiness. (These effects may be less severe than similar effects caused by older sleeping pills.) Not everyone experiences all of these effects.

Conditions in which zolpidem should be avoided

Severe breathing or chest problems, sleep apnoea (a condition where a person spasmodically stops breathing whilst asleep). Myasthenia (a condition in which a person is susceptible to being abnormally fatigued). Serious liver disease or impairment.

Conditions in which zolpidem should be used with caution

Caution is advised in people suffering from depression or with kidney or liver disease. People with a history of drug or alcohol dependence may be at risk of becoming dependent on this drug.

Use in pregnancy and breast-feeding

Zolpidem should not be used during pregnancy or whilst breast-feeding.

ZOPICLONE

Trade name	Description
Zimovane	7.5 mg off-white oval tablets indented with ZM on one side.

General information

Zopiclone is another of the newer tranquillisers prescribed for insomnia. Its effects are similar but different to the older benzo-diazepine sleeping pills. It is said that its side effects are less severe than those of the benzodiazepines. It is a short-acting drug which reduces the risk of its effects persisting into the day following its use but as with all sleeping pills caution is advised in driving. Similarly, it should not be used for more than a few days at a time.

Dosage information

Adult: 7.5 mg at bedtime.
Elderly and physically frail: half the adult dose increased if necessary.
Children: Not recommended for children.

Side effects and further information

Dry mouth, vomiting and stomach upsets. Bitter metallic taste in the mouth. Irritation, confusion and depression. Clumsiness, light headedness and headache. Skin rashes and allergies.

Hallucinations, nightmares, memory problems and aggression. Not everyone experiences all of these effects.

Conditions in which zopiclone should be avoided

Severe liver disease. Severe breathing or chest problems. Sleep apnoea (a condition where a person spasmodically stops breathing whilst asleep). Myasthenia (a condition in which a person is susceptible to being abnormally fatigued).

Conditions in which zopiclone should be used with caution

Caution is advised in people suffering from depression or with kidney or liver disease. People with a history of drug or alcohol dependence may be at risk of becoming dependent on this drug. Caution is also advised in people being treated with other psychiatric drugs. Elderly or frail people should also be cautious about using zopiclone.

Use in pregnancy and breast-feeding

Zopiclone should not be used during pregnancy or whilst breast-feeding.

The Barbiturates

There is no place in treatment of anxiety or insomnia for any of the barbiturate compounds, except for a diminishing number of elderly people who have been maintained on them for many years. The only reason that such patients are maintained on these dangerous drugs is the fact that it would now be too dangerous to attempt to wean them off the drugs. Despite the fact the number of prescriptions for barbiturates has steadily declined over the past 30 years, they continue to kill more people Britain than any other drug. Barbiturates are more dangerous than heroin. Their side effects are worse and their withdrawal effects can be fatal. The barbiturates have a small but problematical role in the control of epilepsy and they are used in anaesthesia. They occupy the somewhat dubious position of being the drug of choice for suicide, for which they are extremely effective. No responsible doctor would prescribe barbiturates for anxiety or insomnia to a patient not already addicted to them.

BARBITURATE TRANQUILLISERS
AND SEDATIVES

Trade name	Description
Amytal	30 mg white tablets marked T56. 50 mg white tablets marked T37. 100 mg white tablets marked T32. 200 mg white tablets marked U13.
Seconal Sodium	50 mg orange capsules marked F42. 100 mg orange capsules marked F40.
Sodium Amytal	60 mg blue capsules marked F23. 60 mg white tablets marked U43. 200 mg blue capsules marked F33. 200 mg white tablets marked U16.
Soneryl	100 mg pink tablets.
Tuinal	100 mg orange/blue capsules marked F65.

General information

Barbiturates should only be prescribed to patients who have been treated with them for a considerable length of time and for whom it is impossible to stop prescribing them because of the risks associated with withdrawal. In effect, they are now used for the maintenance of addicted patients. These compounds are controlled under the provisions of the Misuse of Drugs Regulations, 1985.

Dosage information

Elderly chronic users already hooked on these drugs only.
Amytal: 100–200 mg at bedtime.
Seconal Sodium: 50–100 mg at bedtime.
Sodium Amytal: 60–200 mg at bedtime.
Soneryl: 100–200 mg at bedtime.
Tuinal: 100–200 mg at bedtime.

Side effects and further information

Elderly people are particularly vulnerable to the side effects of these drugs, but at the same time they are more likely to be taking them than anyone else, apart from addicts, amongst whom they are very popular. Elderly people metabolise drugs much more slowly than younger people, which can lead to the drug building up in their bodies to dangerous and potentially fatal levels.

Side effects include: Drowsiness. Lightheadedness. Confusion. Ataxia (shaky movements and unsteady gait caused by the brain's failure to control the body's posture and the strength and direction of limb movements). Impaired memory. Headaches. Vertigo. Dry mouth. Stomach upsets. Reduced urination. Agranulocytosis (a serious deficiency of white blood cells caused by damage to the bone marrow). Allergic reactions. Convulsions. Paradoxically, excitement. Paraesthesia (pins and needles). Tolerance to the effects of the drug. Addiction.

Withdrawal
The withdrawal effects of barbiturate compounds may be sufficiently severe to be life-threatening if left untreated. The effects are: Anxiety. Feelings of weakness. Tension. Loss of appetite. Epileptic fits. Delirium. Hallucinations. According to a standard psychiatric textbook by Slater and Roth (1969), when barbiturates were withdrawn after chronic intoxication 'an acute withdrawal psychosis clinically resembling delirium tremens with anxiety and terrifying hallucinations occurred in three out of five cases, two or three days after admission to hospital'.

Conditions in which barbiturates should be avoided
Barbiturates should not be used at all for anxiety and insomnia, but they are even more dangerous in people who have: porphyria (a rare blood disorder which causes severe sensitivity to sunlight resulting in inflammation or blistering of the skin, inflammation of the nerves, mental disturbances, attacks of stomach pain and blue urine).

Use in pregnancy and breast-feeding
Avoid completely.

PART TWO

Antidepressants

Depression

We use the word 'depressed' to convey to others that we feel sad or unhappy. We may be depressed about losing a job, because of a bereavement or as a consequence of any distressing event in our lives, although sometimes we feel depressed for no obvious reason. (Winston Churchill called the bouts of depression he suffered throughout his adult life his 'black dog'.) But when do these emotions amount to a depression meriting treatment? The simple answer is when extreme sadness, pessimism and despair dominate a person's consciousness and behaviour for an intolerable length of time. Most of us recover from our depression with time and the help of those around us, but some others just seem to sink still further into despair. When this happens and they seek the help of their doctors they are likely to be diagnosed as depressed.

Some people are diagnosed as suffering 'reactive' depression, meaning that it is a reaction to distressing circumstances, others as suffering from 'endogenous' depression, meaning that their depression appears not to have any external cause, and is thus assumed to come from within the sufferer. Not everyone agrees that it is useful or even possible to draw such distinctions, although some drug manufacturers claim their products to be particularly beneficial for one or other of these categories.

Clinical depression

Depression becomes 'clinical' when it has been diagnosed as such by a doctor. Clinical depression is not a specific illness but a term used for a set of symptoms and signs which doctors judge to be serious enough to require treatment. As for the actual causes of these symptoms, however, the term 'clinical' adds nothing to our understanding of them. There are many theories about the nature and causes of depression and although research points to some convincing factors, there is no single cause. Depression is not something that can be caught, like influenza or chickenpox, and neither is it caused by delinquent brain cells or genes, although in some circumstances these may play a part. Depression is the culmination of changes occurring in the mind, body and life of the sufferer. It can be effectively relieved by drugs, but there is no drug which cures it. The good news is that about 60 per cent of people who suffer depression get better, with or without treatment.

Symptoms or signs of 'clinical' depression

Changes in mood: Feelings of gloom and pessimism. Feelings of sadness which are impossible to shake off. A deep sense of personal isolation – feeling cut off from surroundings and other people. These feelings are usually more intense early in the morning or late at night.

Guilt: Nagging feelings of guilt, worthlessness and shame. Sometimes very severely depressed people develop strange ideas and fixed beliefs about themselves or others to the point where they lose contact with reality. They may see, hear, smell or feel touched by things that are not really there. This may be called psychotic depression.

Problems with sleep: Difficulty in getting off to sleep because of persistent fears and anxiety. Sleep becomes fitful, with bouts of restlessness and agitation. Waking up very early in the morning feeling anxious, unrested and drained.

Problems with work and activities: Feeling increasingly unable to cope with the daily demands of work. Continual anxiety, leading to increasing difficulties in making even the simplest decisions and feeling plagued by doubt over any decision made. Everything seems to require more and more effort and less seems to be achieved or achievable. Loss of interest and loss of will. This may lead to a gradual withdrawal from daily activities and contact with other people.

Agitation and anxiety: Anxiety becomes persistent, which may lead to agitation and explosions of rage which are often followed by bouts of extreme remorse.

Slowing down: Thought processes become sluggish and concentration becomes increasingly difficult. The limbs and body feel heavier and require more effort to move. Memory becomes less reliable. Feeling apathetic and increasingly driven inward into the self.

Morbid thoughts and ideas: Obsessive concern or preoccupation with physical health. Minor aches and pains become major worries. Sometimes a fixed belief in an undiagnosed illness. Feelings of unreality, detachment and isolation.

Physical signs and symptoms: Indigestion, wind, constipation, loss of appetite and feelings of heaviness in the stomach. Headaches. Palpitations or heart flutters. Over-breathing. Backache. Muscular aches and pains. Lethargy and persistent fatigue. Reduced sexual arousal, premature ejaculation, impotence, inability to reach orgasm. Periods may become irregular, occurring more or less frequently than usual. Period pains may be more severe and the periods heavier. Loss of weight.

Suicidal ideas: A preoccupation with suicidal thoughts, ideas and speculations which may be acted upon.

Each year more than eight million prescriptions for antidepressants are dispensed in Britain. Estimates as to the proportion of adults in the population diagnosed as clinically depressed vary between two and fifteen per hundred. The large gap between these lower and higher estimates is explained in part by the fact that some doctors are more likely to diagnose it than others. Studies have shown a social-class bias in the way that depression is diagnosed, with middle-class people more likely to be diagnosed as suffering from anxiety or stress, and working-class people more likely to be diagnosed as depressed.

One very striking feature about depression is the fact that women are twice as likely as men to be diagnosed as depressed. The difference in the rates cannot be explained by hormonal or other gender-related physical factors. Premenstrual problems, postnatal depression and the menopause play very small parts in the overall figures.

A gender-related difference which may help to explain women's increased likelihood of suffering depression is the different ways in which the sexes deal with emotional distress. Men are twice as likely as women to become alcoholic or drug abusers, a type of behaviour which may represent a form of 'self-medication'. Such an explanation fits very neatly with the finding that women are more likely than men to seek help from their doctors. Thus, while men are more likely to be seen in the pub when they are low, women are more likely to be seen in the GP's waiting room. Men are substantially more prone to committing crimes, particularly violent crimes. Again, this fits with the view that men tend to externalise their feelings through aggressive behaviour, whilst women tend to internalise them by becoming anxious or depressed.

A broader, socio-economic perspective may also shed some light on women's apparent increased vulnerability to depression. One of the key features of the experience of depression is a feeling of powerlessness. An interesting recent research finding which may have some bearing here is one which suggests that people who are prone to depression are more likely to have a realistic view of life than those who are not. And in a world in which patriarchy in its many forms is prevalent, the objective reality is that women exercise less power in society than men.

A research study done amongst women in Camberwell, South London, showed that about a quarter of working-class women living with children suffered from depression. Amongst these a large proportion would have been diagnosed by a doctor as suffering from depression serious enough to warrant medication or admission to hospital. The rate amongst middle-class women in the same area was 6 per cent. Of the depressed working-class women, most had experienced a serious problem in the previous year, such as the loss of a husband or serious financial problems. However, research into problems such as depression seldom includes the broader socio-economic issues which have such a bearing on the lives of the subjects of that research. Much of it focuses narrowly on personal problems or responses to treatment with drugs. One of the great difficulties of research into mental health is that it seldom looks at the world in which mental ill health occurs. But perhaps there is a risk that we might discover things that we would rather not know about?

Tricyclic antidepressants

The term tricyclic refers to the molecular structure of these drugs which comprises three linked rings of molecules, although not all the antidepressants which are usually classified as tricyclics have this structure. Some in fact have more or less than three molecules. The actual distinctions between them are relatively unimportant, however, as regardless of the way the ingredients are combined, in their effects and side effects, most of these drugs have more similarities than differences. Despite the claims made for these products by their manufacturers the practical differences between them was of little more importance to the consumer than the differences between competing brands of petrol, washing powder or baked beans.

The first of the tricyclic antidepressants was imipramine, which was introduced in 1957 and was followed soon after by amitriptyline. Since then many new products have been added to the tricyclic group, although it appears that doctors maintain some degree of scepticism about the advantages claimed for the newer or second-generation tricyclic antidepressants. Amitriptyline and imipramine remain the most widely prescribed drugs in the group. Newer drugs like the selective serotonin re-uptake inhibitors do appear to have advantages over the tricyclics in that they appear to be as effective with fewer dangerous side effects. They are however considerably more expensive to prescribe.

How effective are tricyclic antidepressants?

Tricyclic antidepressants are effective in reducing the symptoms of depression and can therefore make life more bearable for many people. But they do not work for everyone, and little is actually known about how or why they work. Between 65 and 70 per cent of people who have been diagnosed as suffering from depression can expect to feel less depressed within two to four weeks of starting treatment with a tricyclic antidepressant. Thirty per cent, however, will feel better if they are given a placebo, that is, a dummy drug with no active ingredients whatsoever and possibly containing nothing more potent than chalk or sugar. A review of the controlled studies into the effectiveness of tricyclic antidepressants reveals that more than a third of all such studies showed the active drugs to have been no more effective than the placebos. Nevertheless, whatever the scientific facts, the truth is that many thousands of depressed people feel less depressed when they take them. Whether and to what extent this improvement is due to what medical researchers call the 'placebo effect', or even to old-fashioned magic, is less important than the fact that for many people these drugs are the only means available to them to relieve the misery of their depression.

Side effects – A cause for concern

All medicines have their disadvantages and side effects. The old saying 'No pain no gain', despite its puritan echoes, is well borne in mind when considering treatment with antidepressants. The side effects of antidepressant drugs can be, and often are, severe, so much so that less than half of all prescribed antidepressants are actually taken. Most of them are either thrown away or abandoned in medicine cabinets as dangerous half-forgotten hoards. When asked, the main reason people give for not persevering with their treatment is that they find the side effects of antidepressants intolerable. These can be particularly severe during the early stages of treatment, before any benefit is felt from taking the drug. It can take up to four weeks before the symptoms of the depression are reduced, and during this time many people will feel worse and often more depressed than they did before they started taking the drug. In these circumstances it is not surprising that so many simply stop taking them. However, the combination of the early side effects and the late benefits of these drugs can have tragic consequences.

In Britain at least 300 people take their lives each year using a tricyclic antidepressant, often in combination with tranquillisers or alcohol. The medical profession seems rather sanguine about this death toll. The consensus in the medical literature seems to attribute the deaths simply to the fact that those who died were depressed and therefore by definition suicidal. This sounds uncomfortably like blaming the victim. It avoids the issues raised about the quality of care that is available to people suffering from severe mental distress. These deaths should raise serious issues for those responsible for planning and running our health service.

The over-prescription of benzodiazepines like Valium, Ativan and Mogadon pointed towards major problems in the quality of our mental health services. For example, in Britain the average length of a consultation with a general practitioner is said to be six and a half minutes; the average length of a consultation with a psychiatrist, ten minutes. A survey done by MIND[1] and the BBC *That's Life!* programme amongst more than two thousand long-term tranquilliser users revealed that over 77 per cent had seen their doctors for less than 15 minutes when they were first prescribed tranquillisers. Sixty-eight per cent were not given any information about the drugs they were prescribed. Less than half that were even told they were being prescribed a tranquilliser. Over 47 per cent of those surveyed had received treatment from a psychiatric hospital and of those two-thirds described their psychiatric treatment as being of no help or as being positively harmful. At the time of their first prescriptions a quarter of the survey were given prescriptions for more than one mood-altering drug; by the time they received their sixth the proportion of people prescribed more than one mood-altering drug had risen to half the sample.

The majority of people with serious depression who seek the help of their doctors will be offered a prescription for a tricyclic antidepressant. Some will take the drug as an important part of a treatment programme individually tailored to their needs which their doctors regularly review with them. In these circumstances the drugs are most likely to be effective. Many people will not be so fortunate. They will get little more than repeat prescriptions for the drugs for as long as they continue to collect them. In these circumstances the real value of the tricyclic antidepressants is questionable.

Getting the most from tricyclic antidepressants

Depression is a life-diminishing and sometimes life-threatening condition. The decision to begin a course of medical treatment should be regarded as a major life event for the individual, the family and those closest to him or her. Quite often when a person is seriously depressed he or she is unable or reluctant to consider the pros and cons of embarking on a course of treatment and in such circumstances a husband, wife or friend may wish to share in the decision-making process. In order for that process to be meaningful it must be as informed as possible. A knowledge of side effects may be of crucial importance to all concerned. Those around the depressed person may need to reassure him or her

[1] Lacey, R. and Woodward, S.: *That's Life! Survey on Tranquillisers*. BBC Publications, London, 1985.

that any strange new feelings and discomforts are caused by the drug rather than by a deterioration of his or her mental state. They may also wish to reassure him or her that these side effects may become less troublesome and that some relief can be expected in time. If the drug does not bring relief within an acceptable period, about eight weeks, they may support the individual in seeking an alternative form of treatment. When the time comes to stop taking the drug they may give help and support during the withdrawal period.

Eight-point guide to getting the most from tricyclic antidepressants

1. Tricyclic antidepressants do not cure depression but they do provide effective relief from most of it symptoms for most people who have them appropriately prescribed. A significant minority – between 30 and 40 per cent – will get no benefit from them.
2. The side effects of this group of drugs can be severe, particularly at the outset of treatment and until they begin to diminish the feelings of depression.
3. Antidepressants are extremely dangerous in overdose.
4. It is important that tricyclic drugs are taken as and when they are prescribed. In some circumstances it is advisable that someone close to the depressed person takes charge of the medication, rather than leaving the person with large quantities of pills.
5. The need for the antidepressant to be continued should be reviewed with the doctor at least every six months.
6. Whilst tricyclic antidepressants are not addictive they do have withdrawal effects. If the antidepressant has been taken for more than a few days the drug should not be suddenly stopped but the dose should be gradually reduced over a period of at least 12 weeks.
7. Most depressed people get better in time with or without treatment.
8. Treatment with drugs can be an important step towards eventual recovery but *it is equally important that the social and emotional circumstances in which the person became depressed be reviewed and possibly changed if a lasting recovery is to be achieved.*

FAST FACTS ABOUT
TRICYCLIC ANTIDEPRESSANTS

Purpose?	Treatment of depression.
How do I take the drug?	Tablets or syrup.
When do I take it?	As directed by your doctor.
How long does it take to work?	Between two and four weeks.
Should I expect to experience side effects?	Yes, particularly when you first start taking the drug, but many people find that they become less troublesome as time passes.
What are the most common side effects?	Dry mouth; tiredness; reduced sexual feelings; less frequent urination; constipation; blurred vision; trembling hands; increased appetite; a craving for sweet foods.
What should I do if I experience other distressing side effects?	Notify your doctor.
How long should I continue to take the drug?	This will depend on your needs and circumstances but at least every six months you should review the need to continue with the drug with your doctor.
Is it addictive?	It depends what you mean by addiction!
	If you have taken the antidepressant for more than a month you are likely to experience withdrawal effects. You should withdraw from this drug by a gradual reduction in the dose taken over a period of at least eight weeks.
Can I drive whilst taking it?	Antidepressants will affect your ability to drive safely.
Can I drink alcohol whilst taking it?	If you drink alcohol it will interact with the drug and further impair your ability to drive. It may make you feel ill.

NEVER EXCEED THE PRESCRIBED DOSE • ALWAYS INFORM ANY DENTIST, DOCTOR OR ANAESTHETIST WHO TREATS YOU THAT YOU ARE TAKING THIS DRUG • KEEP MEDICINES OUT OF THE REACH OF CHILDREN.

AMITRIPTYLINE

Trade name	Description
Under generic name	Injection.
Under generic name	10 mg coated tablet.
	25 mg coated tablet.
	50 mg coated tablet.
Lentizol	25 mg pink capsules.
	50 mg pink and red capsules.
Tryptizol	10 mg blue tablets.
	25 mg yellow tablets.
	50 mg brown tablets.
	Pink syrup containing 10 mg per 5 ml.

NEVER EXCEED THE PRESCRIBED DOSE • ALWAYS INFORM ANY DENTIST, DOCTOR OR ANAESTHETIST WHO TREATS YOU THAT YOU ARE TAKING THIS DRUG • KEEP MEDICINES OUT OF THE REACH OF CHILDREN.

General information

One of the first and most commonly prescribed tricyclic antidepressants. Effective for the treatment of depression in about 65 to 70 per cent of people who have been correctly diagnosed. It takes between two and four weeks before the antidepressant effects are felt.

Dosage information

Adult (16 and over): Treatment begins with 50–75 mg daily in divided doses or preferably in a single dose at bedtime, increased gradually if necessary to **a maximum of 150–200 mg per day**. The usual maintenance dose is 50–100 mg per day.

Elderly, physically frail and adolescent: Initially 25–50 mg, increased with caution and close medical supervision to **a maximum of 150 mg per day**.

Children: Amitriptyline is not recommended for the treatment of depression in children below the age of 16. Amitriptyline causes urinary retention and for this reason is sometimes used as a treatment for bedwetting in children. This is an increasingly controversial treatment for bedwetting as it exposes children to unpleasant drug side effects. The treatment works only for as long as the drug is taken. Psychological treatments are more effective and less harmful.

DOSE OF AMITRIPTYLINE USED IN THE TREATMENT OF BEDWETTING

Age of child and body weight	Daily dose
6–10 years (20–35 kg/44–77 lb)	10–20 mg
11–16 years (35–54 kg/77–119 lb)	25–50 mg

OVERDOSE EXTREMELY DANGEROUS • SEEK IMMEDIATE MEDICAL HELP

Side effects and further information See p. 49.

AMOXAPINE

Trade name	Description
Asendis	25 mg white hexagonal tablets marked LL25.
	50 mg orange hexagonal tablets marked LL50.
	100 mg blue hexagonal tablets marked LL100.
	150 mg white hexagonal tablets marked LL150.

NEVER EXCEED THE PRESCRIBED DOSE • ALWAYS INFORM ANY DENTIST, DOCTOR OR ANAESTHETIST WHO TREATS YOU THAT YOU ARE TAKING THIS DRUG •. KEEP MEDICINES OUT OF THE REACH OF CHILDREN.

General information

Amoxapine is closely related to the so-called major tranquillisers and has similar effects and side effects to other tricyclic antidepressants. It can relieve the symptoms of depression within four to seven days of beginning the treatment, as compared to many tricyclic antidepressants which can take between two and four weeks to bring relief. Until the benefits of the drug begin to be felt side effects may cause more problems and the depression may grow worse.

Dosage information

Adult (16 and over): Initially 100–150 mg daily in divided doses or, preferably, in a single dose at bedtime, to be increased gradually if necessary to **a maximum of 300 mg daily.** The usual maintenance dose is 150–250 mg per day.

Elderly and physically frail: Treatment begins with 25 mg twice daily, to be increased if necessary after five to seven days **to a maximum of 50 mg three times daily.**

Children: Amoxapine is not recommended for children.

Overdose extremely dangerous • Seek immediate medical help

Side effects and further information

Women may experience irregular periods and milk may be secreted from their breasts. In long-term use there is a risk of developing a condition called tardive dyskinesia which causes involuntary movements in the mouth, face, trunk and limbs. This condition may be permanent. For a fuller description and discussion of tardive dyskinesia, see pp. 129–130. For further information, see p. 49.

CLOMIPRAMINE

Trade name	Description
Anafranil	10 mg yellow and brown capsules.
	25 mg orange and brown capsules.
	50 mg blue and brown capsules.
	75 mg pink tablets.
	Orange-coloured and flavoured syrup containing 25 mg per ml.
	Injection.
Under generic name	10 mg tablets.
	25 mg tablets.
	50 mg tablets.

NEVER EXCEED THE PRESCRIBED DOSE • ALWAYS INFORM ANY DENTIST, DOCTOR OR ANAESTHETIST WHO TREATS YOU THAT YOU ARE TAKING THIS DRUG • KEEP MEDICINES OUT OF THE REACH OF CHILDREN.

General information

Clomipramine is similar in its effects and side effects to other tricyclic antidepressants and thus probably has no obvious benefits or disadvantages over such drugs as amitriptyline. It is claimed to have benefits for phobias and obsessions when used alongside other treatments. It is also claimed to be useful in the treatment of narcolepsy, a condition in which people tend to fall asleep in quiet surroundings or whilst engaged in monotonous activities. It may take between two and four weeks before the symptoms of depression are relieved. During this time side effects may cause more problems and the feelings of depression may become worse.

Dosage information

Adults (16 and over): Treatment begins with 10 mg daily, to be increased if necessary to **a maximum dose of 150 mg per day**.

The usual maintenance dose is 30–150 mg daily in divided doses or as a single dose at bedtime.

Elderly and physically frail: maximum recommended daily dose is 75 mg.

Children: Not recommended for the treatment of children.

Overdose extremely dangerous • Seek immediate medical help

Side effects and further information See p. 49.

DESIPRAMINE

Trade name	Description
Pertofran	25 mg pale apricot-pink tablets marked EW.

NEVER EXCEED THE PRESCRIBED DOSE • ALWAYS INFORM ANY DENTIST, DOCTOR OR ANAESTHETIST WHO TREATS YOU THAT YOU ARE TAKING THIS DRUG • KEEP MEDICINES OUT OF THE REACH OF CHILDREN.

General information
Desipramine has similar effects and side effects to other tricyclic antidepressants but is said to be less likely to cause drowsiness. It may take between two and four weeks before the symptoms of depression are relieved. During this time the side effects are most likely to cause problems and the feelings of depression may be made worse.

Dosage information
Adult (16 and over): Treatment begins with 75 mg daily in divided doses or as a single dose at bedtime, to be gradually increased if necessary to **a maximum dose of 200 mg**.

Elderly and physical and frail: Initially 25 mg daily, to be gradually increased if necessary.

Children: Not recommended for children.

Overdose extremely dangerous • Seek immediate medical help

Side effects and further information See p. 49.

DOTHIEPIN

Trade name	Description
Prothiaden	25 mg red and brown capsules.
	75 mg red tablets.

NEVER EXCEED THE PRESCRIBED DOSE • ALWAYS INFORM ANY DENTIST, DOCTOR OR ANAESTHETIST WHO TREATS YOU THAT YOU ARE TAKING THIS DRUG • KEEP MEDICINES OUT OF THE REACH OF CHILDREN.

General information

One of the antidepressants with more sedative properties, it can aid sleep or cause drowsiness. Like many of the antidepressants in this group it may take between two and four weeks to relieve the symptoms of depression.

Dosage information

Adult (16 and over): Treatment begins with 75 mg in divided doses or preferably as a single dose at bedtime, to be increased if necessary to **a maximum dose of 150 mg per day.** Patients in hospital may receive up to 200 mg per day.
Elderly and physically frail: Treatment begins with 50–75 mg per day, to be increased, if necessary to **a maximum of 75 mg.**
Children: Not recommended for children.

Overdose extremely dangerous • Seek immediate medical help

Side effects and further information See p. 49.

DOXEPIN

Trade name	Description
Sinequan	10 mg orange capsules.
	25 mg orange and blue capsules.
	50 mg blue capsules.
	75 mg yellow and blue capsules.

NEVER EXCEED THE PRESCRIBED DOSE • ALWAYS INFORM ANY DENTIST, DOCTOR OR ANAESTHETIST WHO TREATS YOU THAT YOU ARE TAKING THIS DRUG • KEEP MEDICINES OUT OF THE REACH OF CHILDREN.

General information

Doxepin has similar effects and side effects to other antidepressants but is more sedating. It can aid sleep or cause drowsiness.

Doxepin is also prescribed for bedwetting in children. It may take between two and four weeks before the symptoms of depression are relieved.

Dosage information
Adult (16 and over): Treatment begins with 75 mg per day in three divided doses. Doses of 100 mg or less per day may be taken as a single dose at bedtime. If necessary the dose may be increased gradually to **a maximum of 300 mg per day**.
Elderly and physically frail: Treatment begins with 10–50 mg per day and is increased gradually with caution. Many elderly people are likely to require no more than 30–50 mg per day.
Children: Not recommended for children under the age of 12.

Overdose extremely dangerous • Seek immediate medical help

Side effects and further information See p. 49.

IMIPRAMINE

Trade name	Description
Under generic name	10 mg tablets.
	25 mg tablets.
Tofranil	10 mg red-brown tablets.
	25 mg red-brown triangular tablets.
	Syrup containing 25 mg per 5 ml.

NEVER EXCEED THE PRESCRIBED DOSE • ALWAYS INFORM ANY DENTIST, DOCTOR OR ANAESTHETIST WHO TREATS YOU THAT YOU ARE TAKING THIS DRUG • KEEP MEDICINES OUT OF THE REACH OF CHILDREN.

General information
The first antidepressant manufactured and one of the more commonly prescribed, its effects and side effects are similar to other tricyclics but it is said to be less sedating. Imipramine is also prescribed for bedwetting in children. It takes between two and four weeks before any relief from symptoms is felt. During this time the side effects are most likely to be a problem and increase the feelings of depression.

Dosage information
Adult (16 and over): Treatment begins with 75 mg per day in divided doses, to be increased gradually to **a maximum of**

200 mg per day. Hospital patients may receive higher doses. Daily doses of 150 mg or less may be taken as a single dose at bedtime.

Elderly and physically frail (60 and over): Treatment begins with 10 mg at night, increased if necessary with caution and close supervision to 10–25 mg three times a day. **Maximum dose is 75 mg per day.**

Children: Not recommended for the treatment of depression in children. Use in bedwetting only. This is a controversial approach to bedwetting. Imipramine only treats the physical side of the problem and exposes child to unpleasant side effects. There are effective psychological treatments for bedwetting.

DOSE OF IMIPRAMINE USED IN THE TREATMENT OF BEDWETTING

Age of child and body weight	Daily dose
6–7 years (20–25 kg/44–55 lb)	25 mg before bedtime.
8–11 years (25–35 kg/55–77 lb)	25–50 mg before bedtime.
Over 11 years (35–54 kg/77–119lb)	50–75 mg bedtime.

Overdose extremely dangerous • Seek immediate medical help

Side effects and further information See p. 49.

LOFEPRAMINE

Trade name	Description
Gamanil	75 mg round brownish-violet tablets.

NEVER EXCEED THE PRESCRIBED DOSE • ALWAYS INFORM ANY DENTIST, DOCTOR OR ANAESTHETIST WHO TREATS YOU THAT YOU ARE TAKING THIS DRUG • KEEP MEDICINES OUT OF THE REACH OF CHILDREN.

General information
One of the newer antidepressants and said to have milder side effects than older drugs. In comparison with other drugs in this group lofepramine does not appear to be substantially more effective. It takes between two and four weeks from the start of treatment before any relief from symptoms is felt. During this time the side effects are most likely to be a problem and increase the feelings of depression.

Dosage information

Adult (16 and over): Between 140–210 mg per day in divided doses. The drug data sheet suggests that in severe cases of depression the doctor may prescribe higher doses on a try-it-and-see basis.

Elderly and physically frail: Lower doses are suggested for elderly people but these are not specified.

Children: The drug data sheet does not specify dose rates for children.

Overdose extremely dangerous • Seek immediate medical help

Side effects and further information

Said to be less severe than the older range of tricyclics. For further information, See p. 49.

MAPROTILINE

Trade name	Description
Ludiomil	25 mg greyish-red tablets marked DP.
	50 mg light orange tablets marked ER.
	75 mg brownish-orange tablets marked ES.

NEVER EXCEED THE PRESCRIBED DOSE • ALWAYS INFORM ANY DENTIST, DOCTOR OR ANAESTHETIST WHO TREATS YOU THAT YOU ARE TAKING THIS DRUG • KEEP MEDICINES OUT OF THE REACH OF CHILDREN.

General information

A 'tetracyclic' antidepressant whose effects and side effects are broadly similar to those of tricyclic drugs. It is said that maprotiline may relieve the symptoms of depression more quickly than many of the antidepressants in this group, i.e. in two to three weeks. It can cause drowsiness and may help to induce sleep.

Dosage information

Adult (16 and over): Treatment begins with 25–75 mg per day in three divided doses or as a single dose at bedtime. Increase if necessary with careful monitoring to **a maximum dose of 150 mg per day**.

Elderly and physically frail: Treatment begins with 10 mg three times per day or a single dose of 30 mg at bedtime. May be increased after one or two weeks to approximately half the normal adult dose.

Children: Not recommended for children.

Overdose extremely dangerous • Seek immediate medical help

Side effects and further information

Skin rashes are not uncommon and people have experienced fits after taking maprotiline. People with a history of epilepsy may be more likely to experience fits but this has also happened to people with no such history. For people suffering from mental disorders which include mania or feelings of persecution this drug may make these symptoms worse. For further information See p. 49.

MIANSERIN

Trade name	Description
Bolvidon	10 mg white tablets marked CT4.
	20 mg white tablets marked CT6.
	30 mg white tablets marked CT7.
Norval	10 mg orange tablets marked 10.
	20 mg orange tablets marked 20.
	30 mg orange tablets marked 30.
Under generic name	10 mg white tablets.
	20 mg white tablets.
	30 mg white tablets.

NEVER EXCEED THE PRESCRIBED DOSE • ALWAYS INFORM ANY DENTIST, DOCTOR OR ANAESTHETIST WHO TREATS YOU THAT YOU ARE TAKING THIS DRUG • KEEP MEDICINES OUT OF THE REACH OF CHILDREN.

General information

The effects and side effects are similar to those of older tricyclic antidepressants. The side effects of mianserin are said to be milder and less common. It exerts a sedative effect which may cause drowsiness or help to induce sleep. For the first three months of treatment the patient's blood should be tested every four weeks for signs of blood or liver disorders. **If the patient develops a fever, sore throat or mouth infection** whilst taking Mianserin the doctor should be notified immediately as this may be a symptom of a potentially dangerous drug reaction.

Dosage information

Adult (16 years and over): Treatment begins with 30–40 mg per day in divided doses or as a single dose at bedtime, increased if necessary to **a maximum dose of 90 mg per day**. The usual main-tenance dose is 30–90 mg per day.

Elderly and physically frail: Treatment begins with up to 30 mg per day, to be increased if necessary under close medical super-vision. Elderly people are often treated with lower than usual doses.

Children: Not recommended for children.

Overdose extremely dangerous • Seek immediate medical help

Side effects and further information
Mianserin is said to have fewer and less frequent side effects than tricyclic antidepressants in general. It is, however, associ-ated with more blood disorders than other drugs and can cause painful swellings in the joints of fingers and toes for a small number of people. For further information See p. 49.

NORTRIPTYLINE

Trade name	Description
Allegron	10 mg white tablets marked DISTA.
	25 mg orange tablets marked DISTA.

NEVER EXCEED THE PRESCRIBED DOSE • ALWAYS INFORM ANY DENTIST, DOCTOR OR ANAESTHETIST WHO TREATS YOU THAT YOU ARE TAKING THIS DRUG • KEEP MEDICINES OUT OF THE REACH OF CHILDREN.

General information
A tricyclic antidepressant with similar effects and side effects to others in the group but said to be less sedating. It takes between two and four weeks from the start of treatment before any relief from symptoms is felt. During this time the side effects are most likely to be a problem and increase the feelings of depression.

Dosage information
Adult (16 and over): Treatment begins with 20–40 mg per day in divided doses or as a single dose at bedtime. Gradually increase if necessary to **a maximum dose of 100 mg per day.** The usual maintenance dose is 30–75 mg per day.

Elderly and physically frail: Treatment begins with 30 mg per day and should be increased with great caution. Elderly people may respond to half the normal adult dose, and may experience side effects more severely.

Children: Not recommended for children as a treatment for depression. Adolescents may be treated for depression with a dose of between 30–50 mg per day in divided doses. Nortriptyline is sometimes controversially used for the treatment of bedwetting. The use of antidepressants exposes children to their potentially serious side effects. Psychological treatments for bedwetting can be more effective.

DOSE OF NORTRIPTYLINE USED IN THE TREATMENT OF BEDWETTING

Age of child and body weight	Daily dose
6–7 years (20–25 kg/44–55 lb)	10 mg
8–11 years (25–35 kg/55–77 lb)	10–20 mg
Over 11 years (35–54 kg/77–119 lb)	25–35 mg

Overdose extremely dangerous • Seek immediate medical help

Side effects and further information
Please note that nortriptyline is said to be less sedating than other drugs in this group. For further information, See p. 49.

PROTRIPTYLINE

Trade name	Description
Concordin	5 mg salmon-pink tablets marked MSD26. 10 mg white tablets marked MSD47.

NEVER EXCEED THE PRESCRIBED DOSE • ALWAYS INFORM ANY DENTIST, DOCTOR OR ANAESTHETIST WHO TREATS YOU THAT YOU ARE TAKING THIS DRUG • KEEP MEDICINES OUT OF THE REACH OF CHILDREN.

General information
One of the many tricyclic antidepressants with similar names and similar effects and side effects. Protriptyline does not cause sedation or drowsiness; in fact, it may have the opposite effect and cause problems with sleep. It takes between two and four

weeks from the beginning of treatment before any relief from symptoms is felt. During this time the side effects are most likely to be a problem and increase the feelings of depression.

Dosage information

Adult (16 and over): Treatment begins with 10 mg three to four times a day, increased if necessary to 60 mg. Once relief from depression is felt the dose should be gradually reduced. If the patient has sleeping difficulties it is recommended that the last dose should be taken before 4 pm. The usual maintenance dose is 15–60 mg per day.

Elderly and physically frail: Treatment begins with 5 mg three times a day, and should be increased with caution and close monitoring of the patient's condition. Doses higher than 20 mg per day increase the risk of the drug causing heart disorders.

Children: Protriptyline is not recommended for children under the age of 16.

Overdose extremely dangerous • Seek immediate medical help

Side effects and further information

Some side effects are more common with protriptyline than with other drugs in this group. These include increased anxiety; agitation; increased heart rate; reduced blood pressure; and increased photosensitivity, resulting in skin rashes after exposure to sunlight. Elderly people are at more risk of experiencing side effects. Of particular concern is the risk of heart damage. For further information See p. 49.

TRAZODONE

Trade name	Description
Molipaxin	50 mg violet and green capsules marked R365B. 100 mg violet and fawn capsules marked R365C. 150 mg pink tablets marked Molipaxin 150. Clear orange-flavoured liquid containing 50 mg per ml.

NEVER EXCEED THE PRESCRIBED DOSE • ALWAYS INFORM ANY DENTIST, DOCTOR OR ANAESTHETIST WHO TREATS YOU THAT YOU ARE TAKING THIS DRUG • KEEP MEDICINES OUT OF THE REACH OF CHILDREN.

General information

Trazodone is not chemically related to the tricyclic antidepressants and appears to have some advantages over many of the drugs in this group. It can relieve the symptoms of depression within one week of beginning the treatment. Trazodone is also said to have fewer and less troublesome side effects. It has strong sedative effects which can cause drowsiness or promote sleep. Alcohol and tranquillisers taken at the same time as trazodone increase the sedative effect.

Dosage information

Adult (16 and over): Treatment begins with 150 mg per day in divided doses after food or as a single dose at bedtime, increased if necessary to **a maximum dose of 300 mg per day**. Patients in hospital may be treated with up to 600 mg per day.

Elderly and physically frail: Treatment begins with 100 mg per day in divided doses after food or as a single dose at bedtime. Increase under supervision to 300 mg per day.

Children: Not recommended for children.

Overdose extremely dangerous • Seek immediate medical help

Side effects and further information

Although trazodone has fewer and less troublesome side effects than other antidepressants, it has on rare occasions caused priapism, a condition in which the penis becomes erect, possibly requiring surgery to return it to normal. For further information See p. 49.

TRIMIPRAMINE

Trade name	Description
Surmontil	10 mg white tablets indented with Surmontil 10.
	25 mg white tablets indented with Surmontil 25.
	50 mg white and green capsules marked SU50.

NEVER EXCEED THE PRESCRIBED DOSE • ALWAYS INFORM ANY DENTIST, DOCTOR OR ANAESTHETIST WHO TREATS YOU THAT YOU ARE TAKING THIS DRUG • KEEP MEDICINES OUT OF THE REACH OF CHILDREN.

General information

Surmontil is similar in its effects and side effects to other tricyclic antidepressants. It has a marked sedative effect which can induce slight drowsiness and promote sleep. It is said that trim-ipramine can relieve the symptoms of depression within seven to ten days. Side effects are usually more pronounced at the beginning of treatment and until the drug has begun to reduce the feelings of depression there is a possibility that the depression may become more pronounced.

Dosage information
Adult (16 and over): 50–75 mg per day taken as a single dose two hours before bedtime, or 25 mg at midday and 50 mg in the evening. Increase if necessary to **a maximum dose of 300 mg per day**. The usual maintenance dose is 75–150 mg per day.
Elderly and physically frail: Treatment begins with 10–25 mg three times per day. It is said that elderly people may benefit with a maintenance dose of half the normal adult dose.
Children: Trimipramine is not recommended for the treatment of children.

Overdose extremely dangerous • Seek immediate medical help

Side effects and further information See opposite.

VILOXAZINE

Trade name	Description
Vivalan	50 mg white tablets marked V.

NEVER EXCEED THE PRESCRIBED DOSE • ALWAYS INFORM ANY DENTIST, DOCTOR OR ANAESTHETIST WHO TREATS YOU THAT YOU ARE TAKING THIS DRUG • KEEP MEDICINES OUT OF THE REACH OF CHILDREN.

General information
Once advertised by its manufacturers as 'the workers' antidepressant', viloxazine is one of the newer antidepressants, said to relieve the symptoms of depression more quickly than many tricyclic antidepressants, and to have fewer and less severe side effects. It does not have a sedative effect; in fact if taken too late in the day it may cause patients difficulty in getting to sleep.

Dosage information
Adult (14 and over): Treatment begins with 300 mg per day, taken 200 mg in the morning and 100 mg at lunchtime. The usual

dose is 300 mg per day, **the maximum dose is 400 mg per day.**
The last dose of the day should not be taken after 6 pm.

Elderly: Treatment begins with 100 mg per day, to be increased
if necessary under close supervision normally to half the adult
dose.

Children: Not recommended for children under the age of 14.

Overdose extremely dangerous • Seek immediate medical help

Side effects and further information

Caution is required for people who suffer from epilepsy, particularly those taking phenytoin. Jaundice and convulsions have
been reported in a small number of people.
For further information, see below.

Tricyclics and related compounds: side effects and further information

Common side effects
Dry mouth. Tiredness. Blurred vision. Constipation. Nausea.
Difficulty in urinating. Weight gain.

Other common side effects
Changes in heart rhythm. Reduced blood pressure leading to
feelings of lightheadedness, sweating, trembling and occasionally fainting. Reduced sexual feelings and difficulty in reaching
orgasm. Men may also have difficulty in achieving or sustaining
an erection. Less commonly some people become alarmingly
excited and confused; these problems are more common in
elderly people and children.

Less common side effects
Black tongue. Obstruction of lower intestine. Epileptic fits.
Agranulocytosis, a potentially fatal blood disorder. Leucopenia,
a dangerous reduction of white blood cells. Eosinophilia, a
blood disorder whose symptoms may include skin rashes and
infections. Purpura and thrombocytopenia, which cause purple
marks on the skin resembling bruising. Jaundice. *Very few
people experience these effects.*

Overdose symptoms
Confusion. Visual hallucinations. Dilated pupils. Reduction in

body temperature. Hyperactivity. Seizure. Stiffening muscles. Coma. Heart failure.

Overdose extremely dangerous • Seek immediate medical help

Withdrawal
Withdrawal from antidepressants should be done over a period of at least four weeks by a gradual reduction of the dose taken. If the drug has been taken for eight weeks or more, under no circumstances should the drug be stopped abruptly. Tricyclic antidepressants are not addictive but many people will experience withdrawal effects when they stop taking them. Withdrawing gradually from the drug gradually will prevent or minimise withdrawal effects.

Withdrawal effects: Nausea. Vomiting. Loss of appetite. Headache. Giddiness. Chills. Less commonly, extreme excitability, insomnia, panic, anxiety and restlessness have been reported.

Conditions in which tricyclic antidepressants must be avoided
Tricyclic antidepressants should not normally be prescribed to people who have had a recent heart attack, suffer from heart disease, are in an extremely excited state, or suffer from porphyria (a rare inherited blood disease).

Conditions in which tricyclic antidepressants should be used with caution
Glaucoma (a condition in which there is high pressure inside the eye). Kidney disease. Epilepsy. Hyperthyroidism and when taking medicine for thyroid disease. Heart disease. Old age. Urination difficulties. They should also be used with caution for people expressing suicidal thoughts, and when receiving electoconvulsive therapy.

Use in pregnancy
Tricyclic antidepressants should be avoided if possible during pregnancy, especially in the first or last three months, unless the depression is life-threatening. Extreme care is needed in balancing the needs of the mother against the risks to the unborn baby.

Use in breast-feeding
Tricyclic antidepressants are carried from mother to baby in the breast milk, which can cause distress to the baby. Increased heart

rates, irritability, muscle spasms and convulsions have been reported in new-born babies of mothers taking tricyclic antidepressants.

Dental damage
Antidepressants inhibit the secretion of saliva and this causes tooth decay, mouth ulcers and changes in the tongue affecting the sense of taste. The dry mouth may persist after the drug has been stopped.

Note: The Committee on the Safety of Medicines has issued a caution in respect of **all** antidepressants concerning a condition called hyponatraemia (a deficiency of sodium in the blood which can cause confusion and drowsiness). This may be a particular problem for elderly people.

HOW TRICYCLIC ANTIDEPRESSANTS INTERACT WITH OTHER DRUGS AND MEDICINES

Drug	Interaction
Alcohol	Alcohol enhances the sedative effects of antidepressants, causing drowsiness.
Other anti-depressants	MAOI antidepressants increase excitability and blood pressure, with potentially dangerous consequences. Fluoxetine increases the level of tricyclic antidepressant compounds in the blood.
Anti-epileptics	The effectiveness of anti-epileptic drugs including barbiturates is reduced and the anti-epileptic drugs themselves reduce the effectiveness of tricyclic antidepressants.
Drugs to reduce blood pressure	The effectiveness of most drugs which reduce blood pressure is enhanced, but in Ismelin, bethanidine, Bendogen, Esbatal, Declinax and clonidine the effectiveness is reduced. There is an increased risk of high blood pressure if clonidine is withdrawn whilst the patient is taking a tricyclic antidepressant.
Antihistimines (commonly found in over-the-counter cold remedies)	Increased sedation which may cause drowsiness.

continued

Drug	Interaction
Antipsychotic drugs (also known as major tranquillisers)	Increased side effects of both drugs (see pp. 125–131), in particular of drugs in the phenothiazine group, such as Largactil.
Tranquillisers and sleeping pills such as Valium, Ativan, Mogadon, etc.	Increased side effects, in particular sedation or drowsiness.
Contraceptive pill and other sex-hormone-based drugs	Sex hormone drugs decrease the positive effects of antidepressants and increase their unpleasant side effects.
Disulfiram. Antabuse, a drug used in the treatment of alcoholism	Increased level of the tricyclic antidepressant in the bloodstream. A potentially dangerous reaction to alcohol may arise if a patient is taking a tricyclic antidepressant at the same time as disulfiram.
Adrenaline, **ephenedrine**, **isoprenaline**, **noradrenaline**. Used in the treatment of heart disease	Potentially dangerous rises in blood pressure and changes in heart rate.
Cimetidine. **Tagamet**, **Dyspamet**, **Algitec**. Used in the treatment of duodenal and gastric ulcers.	Increased levels of antidepressant compounds in the blood stream.
Nitrates. Drugs used to treat angina and heart attacks, such as glyceryl trinitrate, Nitrocine, Nitronal, Tridil etc.	Tricyclic antidpressants cause the mouth to dry, therefore reducing the effectiveness of drugs used to treat angina and heart attack by preventing them from being dissolved in the mouth as quickly

ALWAYS INFORM ANY NEW DOCTOR OR DENTIST WHO IS TREATING YOU THAT YOU ARE TAKING AN ANTIDEPRESSANT.

MAOI antidepressants

Monoamine oxidase inhibitor (MAOI) antidepressants are a second-choice treatment for severely depressed people who fail to benefit from other treatments or treatment with other antidepressants. The name refers to the way they inhibit production of the enzyme which affects the production of 'monoamines', that is adrenaline, noradrenaline and serotonin, and others. The first MAOI antidepressant was iproniazid, which had previously been used as a treatment for tuberculosis. In the late 1940s it was noted that this drug caused elation in TB patients and this led to its being tried as an antidepressant. MAOI antidepressants have had a very chequered history, and a number of them including iproniazid have been withdrawn from use because experience showed them to be dangerous. A significant number of patients treated with MAOIs suffered serious liver damage. Some patients become very agitated, occasionally losing contact with reality and experiencing psychotic episodes.

The major problem with the MAOI antidepressants is that they interact dangerously with certain common foods, drinks and over-the-counter medicines. The foods, drugs and drinks which must be avoided are listed on p. 61. It is extremely important that patients stick to these dietary rules on whilst taking MAOI antidepressants and for at least three weeks after they stop. The dietary problems of these drugs are not, however, the sole reason for concern about their use. Withdrawing from MAOIs is more difficult than from tricyclics because their effects are often much more severe. The frequency of serious side effects is also higher with MAOIs. One study comparing the side effects of phenelzine (an MAOI), imipramine (a tricyclic) and a placebo (a dummy drug), showed that over a period of 33 weeks, 14 per cent of patients treated with the placebo reported a serious side effect, compared with 27 per cent of those on imipramine and 90 per cent of those on phenelzine. Of those treated with phenelzine, 10 per cent experienced a psychotic or near-psychotic episode, 8 per cent experienced a critical rise in blood pressure, 8 per cent had an increase in weight of over 15 pounds and 22 per cent experienced impotence or the inability to reach orgasm. In all, 132 serious side effects were noted for the 141 patients treated with phenelzine in this study. The MAOIs are also extremely dangerous in overdose which is why they are prescribed as a treatment of last resort for depression.

These old MAOIs are now obsolescent. Newer MAOIs are being introduced which seem from early experience to have fewer and less severe problems whilst being as effective as other antidepressants. These are the reversible MAOIs.

FAST FACTS ABOUT MONOAMINE OXIDASE INHIBITOR ANTIDEPRESSANTS

Purpose	Treatment of depression
How do I take it?	As directed by your doctor. If you are uncertain seek the advise of your doctor or pharmacist.
How long does it take to work?	Between two and four weeks.
Should I expect to experience side effects?	Yes, particularly when you first begin to take the drug. Not everyone finds these side effects to be too troublesome, and many find them to become less so as time passes.
What are the most common side effects?	Dry mouth; drowsiness; nausea; headache; fatigue; restlessness; insomnia; constipation; blurred vision; swelling ankles.
What should I do if I experience other distressing side effects?	Notify your doctor at once. If you experience a sudden rise in temperature accompanied by a severe throbbing headache seek urgent medical advice.
How long should I continue to take it?	This will depend on your needs and circumstances but you should review with your doctor your need to continue with the drug at least every six months. If the drug has not relieved your depression after six weeks you are unlikely to obtain any benefit from it.
Can I drive whilst taking it?	Antidepressants will affect your ability to drive safely.
Can I drink alcohol whilst taking it?	You should avoid red wines, lager and non-alcoholic beers. The drug will interact with any alcoholic drink and further impair your ability to drive.
Should I take any special precautions whilst taking it?	Yes, you must be careful to avoid certain foods, drinks, and medicines see the list on p. 61).
Is it addictive?	It all depends what you mean by addiction! You must withdraw from the drug gradually over a period of eight weeks or more in order to minimise its withdrawal effects.

NEVER EXCEED THE PRESCRIBED DOSE • ALWAYS INFORM ANY DOCTOR, DENTIST OR ANAESTHETIST THAT YOU ARE TAKING AN MAOI ANTIDE-PRESSANT • BE CAREFUL ABOUT WHAT YOU EAT AND DRINK AND BE PAR-TICULARLY CAREFUL ABOUT ANY MEDICINES YOU BUY OR ARE PRESCRIBED • KEEP MEDICINES OUT OF THE REACH OF CHILDREN

ISOCARBOXAZID

Trade name	Description
Marplan	10 mg round pink tablets.

General information
Like other drugs in the MAOI group, isocarboxazid is most appropriately prescribed when no other antidepressant or chemical treatment has been effective. For a small number of people MAOIs sometimes bring rapid and pronounced relief from the symptoms of depression. For between 25 and 40 per cent of people they are unlikely to be of any benefit. Side effects are more common and more pronounced than with the tricyclic group of antidepressant drugs.

Dosage information
Adult (16 and over): Treatment begins with 30 mg per day as a single dose or in three doses through the day. If the drug has not relieved the depression the dose may be gradually increased with great care and under close supervision to **a maximum dose of 60 mg per day for a period of no longer than six weeks**. If the depression has not been relieved after this time the drug should gradually be withdrawn as it will be unlikely to have any positive effect. At the higher dose levels there is a greater likelihood of serious side effects. Once the symptoms of the depression have been relieved the dose should gradually be reduced to the lowest level effective in relieving the depression.
Elderly and physically frail: It is recommended that elderly people should be treated at half the adult dose. Elderly people are more likely to suffer from side effects such as confusion, agitation and reduced blood pressure.
Children: Isocarboxazid is not recommended for children.

Side effects and further information
Isocarboxazid, like the other MAOI antidepressants, is most definitely not the first-choice treatment amongst drug options for

the treatment of depression. Its serious side effects and the way in which it interacts with other drugs and certain foods makes it a potentially hazardous treatment. It is said to be less likely to cause liver damage than phenelzine.

See page 61 for list of foods, drinks and over-the-counter medicines which must be avoided whilst taking this drug.

NEVER EXCEED THE PRESCRIBED DOSE • ALWAYS INFORM ANY DOCTOR, DENTIST OR ANAESTHETIST THAT YOU ARE TAKING A MAOI ANTIDE-PRESSANT • BE CAREFUL ABOUT WHAT YOU EAT AND DRINK AND BE PARTICULARLY CAREFUL ABOUT ANY MEDICINES YOU BUY OR ARE PRESCRIBED • KEEP MEDICINES OUT OF THE REACH OF CHILDREN

Overdose extremely dangerous • Seek immediate medical help

MOCLOBEMIDE

Trade name	Description
Manerix	150 mg pale yellow oblong tablet.
	300 mg whitish yellow oblong tablet.

General information

Moclobemide is a new type of MAOI antidepressant which appears to be less hazardous than the older drugs in this group. It works in a similar way to the older drugs but has a more specific and weaker inhibiting effect on the monoamine oxidase enzymes. This means it is less likely to cause the rapid rise in blood pressure and other problems if a patient consumes food, drink or over-the-counter medicines which contain tyramine. However, patients are still advised to observe the dietary guidelines issued with prescriptions for MAOI antidepressants.

Dosage information

Adult (16 and over): Treatment begins with 300 mg per day in divided doses after meals increased or decreased as necessary to achieve the best result. Normal treatment ranges between 150 and 300 mg per day.

Children: Not recommended for children.

Conditions in which moclobemide should be used with caution

People in excited or agitated states of mind. People suffering from manic depressive mood swings. Serious liver disease. Thyrotoxosis (a condition in which excessive thyroid hormones in the bloodstream causes anxiety, sweating, rapid heart beat, sweating, trembling, increased appetite, loss of weight and sensitivity to heat).

Conditions in which moclobemide should not be used

Pregnancy. People in seriously confused states of mind. Phaeochromocytoma (a tumour in the adrenal gland which causes the uncontrolled release of adrenaline and noradrenaline causing increased blood pressure, palpitations, increased heart rate and headache).

Side effects and further information

Moclobemide may cause dizziness, nausea, headache and confusion.

See page 61 for list of foods, drinks and over-the-counter medicines which must be avoided whilst taking this drug

NEVER EXCEED THE PRESCRIBED DOSE • ALWAYS INFORM ANY DOCTOR, DENTIST OR ANAESTHETIST THAT YOU ARE TAKING AN MAOI ANTIDE-PRESSANT • BE CAREFUL ABOUT WHAT YOU EAT AND DRINK AND BE PARTICULARLY CAREFUL ABOUT ANY MEDICINES YOU BUY OR ARE PRESCRIBED • KEEP MEDICINES OUT OF THE REACH OF CHILDREN

Overdose extremely dangerous • Seek immediate medical help

PHENELZINE

Trade name	Description
Nardil	15 mg orange tablets.

General information

Phenelzine is one of the older MAOI antidepressants which are generally regarded as treatments of last resort. It is important that whilst taking this drug and for three weeks after stopping it patients avoid foods and drinks containing tyramine. A card listing foods, drinks and medicines which should be avoided is issued with prescriptions for phenelzine. The benefits of this drug may not be felt for four weeks after it is begun and during this time its side effects can be very severe. If no benefit has been has been achieved after six weeks it is unlikely that any benefit will be achieved from its continued use.

Dosage information

Adult (16 and over): Treatment begins with 15 mg three times per day increased if necessary to 15 mg four times a day after two weeks. The dose should then be slowly reduced until the best result is achieved for the individual patient. Some patients may only need to take one 15 mg tablet on alternate days. Patients in hospital are sometimes given higher doses (up to 30 mg three times per day).
Children: Not recommended for children.

Conditions in which phenelzine should be used with caution

Diabetes, heart disease, epilepsy, and blood disorders. Caution is advised in patients receiving electro-convulsive therapy.

Conditions in which phenelzine should be avoided

Pregnancy, breast-feeding mothers and the elderly. Should also be avoided by patients suffering from porphyria (a rare inherited blood disease which causes periods of mental disturbance).

Side effects and further information

Dry mouth; drowsiness; nausea; headache; fatigue; restlessness; insomnia; constipation; blurred vision; swollen ankles. Phenelzine should not be stopped abruptly but gradually withdrawn over at least eight weeks. **See page 61 for list of foods, drinks and over-the-counter medicines which must be avoided by patients taking this drug.**

NEVER EXCEED THE PRESCRIBED DOSE • ALWAYS INFORM ANY DOCTOR, DENTIST OR ANAESTHETIST THAT YOU ARE TAKING AN MAOI ANTIDEPRESSANT • BE CAREFUL ABOUT WHAT YOU EAT AND DRINK AND BE PARTICULARLY CAREFUL ABOUT ANY MEDICINES YOU BUY OR ARE PRESCRIBED • KEEP MEDICINES OUT OF THE REACH OF CHILDREN

Overdose extremely dangerous • Seek immediate medical help

TRANYLCYPROMINE

Trade name	Description
Parnate	10 mg geranium red tablets marked SKF.

General information

Tranylcypromine is one of the older MAOI antidepressants which are generally regarded as treatments of last resort. Tranylcypromine was formerly described in the British National Formulary as 'the most hazardous of the MAOIs because of its stimulant action.' It is important that whilst taking this drug and for three weeks after stopping it patients avoid foods and drinks containing tyramine. A card listing foods, drinks and medicines which should be avoided is issued with prescriptions for tranylcypromine. The benefits of this drug may not be felt for four weeks after it is begun and during this time its side effects can be very severe. Tranylcypromine is more likely than other MAOIs to cause a rapid and potentially dangerous rise in blood pressure associated with the consumption of foods and drinks containing tyramine. If no benefit has been has been achieved after six weeks it is unlikely that any benefit will be achieved from its continued use.

Dosage information

Adult (16 and over): Treatment begins with 10 mg taken twice a day not later than 3 pm. After one week the second dose may be increased if necessary to 20 mg. Doses over 30 mg per day require considerable thought and close supervision. The usual daily dose is 10 mg per day.
Children: Not recommended for children.

Side effects and further information

Dry mouth; drowsiness; nausea; headache; fatigue; restlessness; insomnia; constipation; blurred vision; swollen ankles. This drug can have a stimulant effect and some patients may become highly agitated or excited. Tranylcypromine should not be stopped abruptly but gradually withdrawn over at least eight weeks.

See page 61 for list of foods, drinks and over-the-counter medicines which must be avoided by patients taking this drug.

NEVER EXCEED THE PRESCRIBED DOSE • ALWAYS INFORM ANY DOCTOR, DENTIST OR ANAESTHETIST THAT YOU ARE TAKING AN MAOI ANTIDE-PRESSANT • BE CAREFUL ABOUT WHAT YOU EAT AND DRINK AND BE PAR-TICULARLY CAREFUL ABOUT ANY MEDICINES YOU BUY OR ARE PRESCRIBED • KEEP MEDICINES OUT OF THE REACH OF CHILDREN

Overdose extremely dangerous • Seek immediate medical help

MAOI antidepressants: side effects and further information

Common side effects
Dizziness. Reduced blood pressure. Blurred vision. Dry mouth. Feelings of weakness. Drowsiness. Constipation. Nausea. Vomiting. Insomnia. Oedema (a retention of bodily fluids which can cause swelling in the legs and ankles). Increased appetite and possibly a craving for sweet foods. Weight gain.

Less common side effects
Headache. Sweating. Convulsions. Feelings of excitement. Neuritis (inflammation of the nerves). Difficulty with urination. Changes in behaviour. Reduced sexual feelings (in men impotence and difficulty in ejaculation). Changes in heart rhythm. Rashes. Trembling hands. Blood disease. Purpura (bruise-like blotches on the skin caused by the rupture of capillaries). Nervousness. Liver damage. Elderly people are more likely to experience these side effects and to experience them more severely.

Symptoms of overdose
Mania. Agitation. Coma. Reduced blood pressure or rapidly increased blood pressure. Bleeding into the brain.

Withdrawal
MAOI antidepressants must be withdrawn over a period of not less than eight weeks by a gradual reduction of the dose. If the drug has been taken for a period of eight weeks or more, under no circumstances should it be stopped abruptly. A gradual withdrawal will prevent or minimise any withdrawal effects.

Withdrawal effects: Nausea. Vomiting. Loss of appetite. Giddiness. Insomnia. Nightmares. Feeling cold. Some people may become extremely agitated and prone to severe panic attacks or mania.

Conditions in which MAOI antidepressants must be avoided

Liver disease. Cerebrovascular diseases (disorders of the blood vessels and membranes of the brain). Phaeochromocytoma (a small tumour in the adrenal gland which causes attacks of raised blood pressure, increased heart rate palpitations and severe headaches). Porphyria (a rare inherited disorder causing skin inflammation or blistering under exposure to sunlight, stomach pains and mental disturbances). Tranylcypromine (Parnate) should not be prescribed to people who suffer from hyperthyroidism.

Children, elderly and agitated people should not be treated with MAOI antidepressants.

Conditions in which MAOI antidepressants should be used with caution

Diabetes. Blood disease.

Use in pregnancy and breast-feeding

MAOI antidepressants should be avoided in pregnancy and during breast-feeding unless the depression constitutes a severe risk to the mother or child and there is no other available form of treatment.

Important dietary precautions when taking MAOI antidepressants

The following is a list of foods, drinks and patent medicines which must be avoided whilst taking MAOI antidepressants:

Cheeses, particularly strong cheeses such as Camembert, Cheddar, Stilton and 'blue' cheeses. Broad bean pods, pickled herrings, yoghurt, bananas, caviar, game (for example, hung pheasant, jugged hare, etc.). Bovril, Marmite, and any similar meat or yeast extracts. Smoked fish, meat and sausages.

Avoid red wines, in particular burgundy, Chianti, sherry and port. Be cautious of all beers, particularly lagers and non-alcoholic beers; some may be hazardous.

Avoid patent medicines sold in chemists and other shops. In particular avoid over-the-counter medicines for the common cold and pain relief such as Nightnurse, Contact 400, Lemsip, Beecham's powders, etc. (Even if you are not taking an MAOI antidepressant these products may only be of marginal value to you and all have their own side effects.)

Always check with your doctor or pharmacist whether a drug is safe for you, whether it is prescribed for you or sold in a shop. This includes inhalants, suppositories, cough sweets, lozenges, nose drops and cough medicines. All of these may be hazardous for you if you take them whilst you are taking an MAOI antidepressant.

Symptoms of the reaction between MAOI drugs and the above foods, drinks and medicines

Very severe throbbing headache, a rapid rise in blood pressure and a very high temperature. If you experience these symptoms whilst taking an MAOI antidepressant seek immediate medical help.

HOW MAOI ANTIDEPRESSANTS INTERACT WITH OTHER DRUGS AND MEDICINES

Drug	Interaction
Pain killers such as codeine, diamorphine, pethidine, dihydrocodeine, methadone. (Diconal, Fortral, Meptid, Narphen, Nubain, Palfium, Temgesic)	Excitement or depression. Increased or decreased blood pressure.
Other MAOI antidepressants	An increase in the side effects and hazards associated with these drugs. (If a patient is to be changed from one MAOI anti-depressant to another, a period of at least ten days should pass between stopping one drug and starting another at a reduced dose.)
Tricyclic antidepressants	Excitability, increase in side effects and possibly an increased risk of potential hazards. Increased blood pressure. It is dangerous to take an MAOI antidepressant at the same time as, or within 14 days of, a tricyclic antidepressant. **The combination of tranylcypromine with clomipramine is very dangerous.**
Tryptophan	Excitability and confusion.
Drugs used to treat diabetes	The effect of insulin and other antidiabetic drugs is enhanced.

continued

Drug	Interaction
Drugs used to treat blood pressure	Enhanced effects of medicines containing reserpine, methyldopa and guanethidine. Excitability and increased blood pressure.
Drugs used to treat epilepsy	MAOI antidepressants decrease the effectiveness of drugs prescribed to reduce convulsions. The manufacturers of carbamazepine (Tegretol) recommend that the drug should not be taken with MAOI antidepressants or used within two weeks of taking an MAOI.
Antimuscarinic drugs such as atropine, used to treat a variety of conditions including Parkinson's disease; Irritable bowel, and others	Increased side effects.
Buspirone (Buspar)	Increased blood pressure. It is recommended that buspirone should not be prescribed for people taking MAOI antidepressants.
Oxypertine (Integrin). Used to treat serious mental distress such as schizophrenia	Excitability and a risk of a dangerous rise in blood pressure.
Levodopa (Brocadopa and Larodopa). Used in the treatment of Parkinson's disease	A serious risk of a dangerous rise in blood pressure.
Sympathomimetic drugs. Adrenaline, noradrenaline, dopamine and isoprenaline. May be present in common cold remedies. Also drugs like amphetamines, used controversially in the treatment of obesity and the control of hyperactive children	Risk of a dangerous increase in blood pressure.
Tetrabenazine (Nitoman). Used to treat tics and other involuntary body movements caused by brain disorders	Excitability and a risk of a dangerous rise in blood pressure.

BE SURE TO INFORM ANY DOCTOR, DENTIST OR ANAESTHETIST TREATING YOU IF YOU ARE TAKING AN MAOI ANTIDEPRESSANT.

Compound antidepressants

Compound antidepressants are tablets which contain mixtures of two drugs. According to the British National Formulary these compounds are not to be recommended because the doses of the ingredient drugs should each be adjusted according to the needs of the individual patient. They contain a mixture of two active drugs, one an antidepressant and the other either an antipsychotic or a minor tranquilliser. Drugs prescribed for depression are usually taken for periods of months or even years which causes particular problems. Compound drugs which contain a minor tranquilliser with the antidepressant present a risk to the patient of becoming addicted to the minor tranquilliser. There is now a clear consensus that minor tranquillisers should not be taken for more than two weeks at a time.

Other compound antidepressants contain an antipsychotic with an antidepressant. These expose patients to enhanced side effects and to the long-term hazards of the antipsychotics. Of particular concern here are two worrying conditions caused by the long-term use of antipsychotics: tardive dyskinesia and dopamine supersensitivity. Tardive dyskinesia causes people to develop involuntary facial tics and other uncontrollable bodily movements (see the section on tardive dyskinesia, pp. 129–130). Dopamine supersensitivity causes people to have psychotic episodes when they reduce or stop their intake of antipsychotic drugs. Both conditions are quite often irreversible. Tardive dyskinesia has been referred to as the stigmata of the modern psychiatric patient.

However, despite the fact that they are not recommended, the following compound antidepressants are apparently available for prescription. For details of their effects and side effects see the chapters describing the effects and side effects of tricyclic antidepressants (p. 49), MAOI antidepressants (p. 60) and antipsychotic drugs (p. 125).

COMPOUND ANTIDEPRESSANT PRODUCTS

Trade name	Description
Triptafen	Pink tablet containing 25 mg of amitriptyline hydrochloride and 2 mg perphenazine.
Triptafen – M	Pink tablet containing 10 mg of amitriptyline hydrochloride and 2 mg perphenazine.

General information
The above pills combine the tricyclic antidepressant amitriptyline with the antipsychotic drug perphenazine.

Trade name	Description
Parstelin	Green tablets containing 10 mg tranylcypromine and 1 mg trifluoperazine.

General information
Parstelin combines the most problematic MAOI antidepressant with an antipsychotic drug.

Selective serotonin re-uptake inhibitors

More hype than miracle
Prozac, or fluoxetine to give it its generic name, is the best known of this relatively new group of antidepressant drugs collectively referred to as SSRIs which act by inhibiting the re-uptake of serotonin or 5-hydroxytryptamine (5-HT) in the brain where it acts as a neurotransmitter. Neurotransmitters are involved in transmitting messages between nerve cells in the brain. Serotonin is widely distributed throughout the body in blood, the walls of the intestine and the central nervous system. The function of serotonin is not fully understood but it appears to have some effects on mood. Prozac has been at the centre of a massive amount of hyperbole in the press and the media. In 1990 it made the cover of *Newsweek* under the banner headline 'A Breakthrough Drug for Depression'. Within two years of its release in 1987 fluoxetine was outselling all other antidepressants on the market in the United States. A certain Doctor Peter Kramer wrote a best-selling book called *Listening to Prozac* in which he coined the term 'cosmetic psychopharmacology'. Kramer suggested that Prozac offered us the opportunity to choose a zippier, more motivated personality out of a bottle. Despite the fact that the author's enthusiasm for the drug far exceeded the evidence he offered for his tantalising propositions, *Listening to Prozac* struck a chord with an enthusiastic public.

Prozac was not without its critics and stories began to emerge in which it was alleged that the drug was behind all sorts of horrors ranging from mass murder to suicide. Prozac's advocates

FAST FACTS ABOUT SSRI ANTIDEPRESSANTS

Purpose	The treatment of depression.
How do I take the drug?	As advised by your doctor. If you are uncertain seek the advice of your doctor or pharmacist.
How long does it take to work?	Between two and four weeks.
When do I take it?	As advised by your doctor.
Should I expect side effects?	Yes, particularly when you first start taking the drug but many people find that any side effects become less troublesome as time passes.
What are the most common side effects?	Gastric upsets, nausea, vomiting, diarrhoea, wind, constipation, loss of appetite and weight loss. Dry mouth, insomnia, headache and anxiety. These effects are dose related. **If you develop a skin rash seek urgent advice from your doctor.**
How long should I continue to take the drug?	This will depend on your needs and circumstances but at least every six months you should review your need to continue with the drug with your doctor.
Is it addictive?	It depends what you mean by addiction!
	You should not stop taking the drug abruptly as you may experience unpleasant withdrawal effects including vaginal bleeding, gastric upsets, sleep disturbances, and anxiety.
Can I drive whilst taking it?	Antidepressants will affect your ability to drive safely.
Can I drink alcohol whilst taking it?	Alcohol will interact with this drug and further impair your ability to drive. If you drink heavily it will make you feel ill.

NEVER EXCEED THE PRESCRIBED DOSE • ALWAYS INFORM ANY DENTIST, DOCTOR OR ANAESTHETIST WHO TREATS YOU THAT YOU ARE TAKING THIS DRUG • KEEP MEDICINES OUT OF THE REACH OF CHILDREN.

and critics pursued their causes with an almost religious zeal – the one side describing it as miracle drug and the other as a devil's brew. The reality behind all this hype is somewhat more mundane. Prozac is not a wonder drug although it is most certainly a very profitable one for its manufacturers. Together with its chemical cousins Prozac is about as effective as the older tricyclic antidepressants. The principle advantages of the SSRIs is that their side effects tend to be less severe and they are considerably less toxic in overdose. Their principle disadvantage compared to the tricyclics is their cost. They are up to ten times more expensive than the most widely prescribed tricyclic antidepressants. Given the toxicity and the side effects of the older drugs the SSRIs appear to have real advantages over them. However, the history of hyped 'safer' drugs is such that it would be wise to temper our enthusiasm for them with caution. Ten or twenty years from now we may take a very different view of the SSRIs.

CITALOPRAM

Trade name	Description
Cipramil	20 mg tablets.

General information
Citalopram is a selective serotonin re-uptake inhibitor antidepressant. It is no more effective than older antidepressant drugs but its side effects are less severe and it is much less toxic in overdose. These factors make it preferable to tricyclic and MAOI antidepressants for most patients.

Dosage information
Adult (16 and over): 20 mg per day taken as a single dose in the morning. This may be increased if necessary to **a maximum dose of 60 mg per day**.
Elderly and physically frail: The maximum dose should not exceed 40 mg per day.
Children: Not recommended for the treatment of children.

Side effects and further information
Citalopram may cause a wide variety of side effects. If a rash develops it is recommended that the drug be stopped as this could be symptomatic of vasculitis (the inflammation of small

blood vessels), anaphylaxis (an allergic reaction), inflammation of the lung or fibrosis (a scarring of tissues following injury or inflammation). Nausea. Vomiting. Diarrhoea. Loss of appetite, leading to weight loss. Headache. Nervousness. Insomnia. Anxiety. Tremors. Dry mouth. Dizziness. Hypomania (elated mood, uninhibited behaviour, rapid speech and abnormal energy). Drowsiness. Convulsions. Fever. Sexual difficulties. Sweating. Less common side effects are blood changes and reduced white blood cell count. Other side effects reported are: Vaginal bleeding after withdrawal of the drug. Anaemia. Thrombocytopenia (a blood disorder which may cause bleeding into the skin, leading to bruise marks and in the event of an injury a tendency to increased bleeding). Confusion.

Use with caution in patients with liver or kidney disease, epilepsy and diabetes. Avoid in pregnancy and in breast-feeding mothers.

It may impair driving ability.

NEVER EXCEED THE PRESCRIBED DOSE • ALWAYS INFORM ANY DENTIST, DOCTOR OR ANAESTHETIST WHO TREATS YOU THAT YOU ARE TAKING THIS DRUG • KEEP MEDICINES OUT OF THE REACH OF CHILDREN.

FLUOXETINE

Trade name	Description
Prozac	20 mg green and off-white capsules.

General information
Fluoxetine is the best known of the selective serotonin re-uptake inhibitor drugs (SSRIs). The publicity which has been focused on this drug has tended to confuse rather than clarify its actual value as a treatment for serious depression. It is no more effective than older antidepressant drugs but its side effects are less severe and it is much less toxic in overdose. These factors make it preferable to tricyclic and MAOI antidepressants for most patients. Time and experience will allow us to reach a better judgement on this over-hyped drug.

Dosage information
Adult (16 and over): For depression, 20 mg per day. For bulima nervosa (an eating disorder), 60 mg per day.

Elderly and physically frail: The maximum dose should not exceed 60 mg per day.

Children: Not recommended for the treatment of children.

Side effects and further information

Fluoxetine may cause a wide variety of side effects. If a rash develops it is recommended that the drug be stopped as this could be symptomatic of vasculitis (the inflammation of small blood vessels), anaphylaxis (an allergic reaction), inflammation of the lung or fibrosis (a scarring of tissues following injury or inflammation). Nausea. Vomiting. Diarrhoea. Loss of appetite, leading to weight loss. Headache. Nervousness. Insomnia. Anxiety. Tremors. Dry mouth. Dizziness. Hypomania (elated mood, uninhibited behaviour, rapid speech and abnormal energy). Drowsiness. Convulsions. Fever. Sexual difficulties. Sweating. Less common side effects are blood changes and reduced white blood cell count. Other side effects reported are: Vaginal bleeding after withdrawal of the drug. Anaemia. Thrombocytopenia (a blood disorder which may cause bleeding into the skin, leading to bruise marks and in the event of an injury a tendency to increased bleeding). Confusion.

Use with caution in patients with liver or kidney disease, epilepsy and diabetes. Avoid in pregnancy and in breast-feeding mothers.

It may impair driving ability.

NEVER EXCEED THE PRESCRIBED DOSE • ALWAYS INFORM ANY DENTIST, DOCTOR OR ANAESTHETIST WHO TREATS YOU THAT YOU ARE TAKING THIS DRUG • KEEP MEDICINES OUT OF THE REACH OF CHILDREN.

FLUVOXAMINE

Trade name	Description
Faverin	50 mg glossy white tablet marked Duphar 291.
	100 mg glossy white tablet marked Duphar 313.

General information

Fluvoxamine is a selective serotonin re-uptake inhibitor antidepressant. It is no more effective than older antidepressant drugs but its side effects are less severe and it is much less toxic in overdose. These factors make it preferable to tricyclic and MAOI antidepressants for most patients. Fluvoxamine may cause slowing of the heart rate.

Dosage information
Adult (16 and over): 100–200 mg per day (taken as a maximum single dose of 100 mg in the evening). This may be increased if necessary to **a maximum dose of 300 mg per day.**
Elderly and physically frail: No special dosage instructions.
Children: Not recommended for the treatment of children.

Side effects and further information
Fluvoxamine may cause a wide variety of side effects. If a rash develops it is recommended that the drug be stopped as this could be symptomatic of vasculitis (the inflammation of small blood vessels), anaphylaxis (an allergic reaction), inflammation of the lung or fibrosis (a scarring of tissues following injury or inflammation). Nausea. Vomiting. Diarrhoea. Loss of appetite, leading to weight loss. Headache. Nervousness. Insomnia. Anxiety. Tremors. Dry mouth. Dizziness. Hypomania (elated mood, uninhibited behaviour, rapid speech and abnormal energy). Drowsiness. Convulsions. Fever. Sexual difficulties. Sweating. Less common side effects are blood changes and reduced white blood cell count. Other side effects reported are: Vaginal bleeding after withdrawal of the drug. Anaemia. Thrombocytopenia (a blood disorder which may cause bleeding into the skin, leading to bruise marks and in the event of an injury a tendency to increased bleeding). Confusion.

Use with caution in patients with liver or kidney disease, epilepsy and diabetes. Avoid in pregnancy and in breast-feeding mothers.

It may impair driving ability.

NEVER EXCEED THE PRESCRIBED DOSE • ALWAYS INFORM ANY DENTIST, DOCTOR OR ANAESTHETIST WHO TREATS YOU THAT YOU ARE TAKING THIS DRUG • KEEP MEDICINES OUT OF THE REACH OF CHILDREN.

NEFAZADONE

Trade name	Description
Dutonin	100 mg white hexagonal tablets marked 100.
	200 mg light yellow hexagonal tablets marked 200.

General information

Nefazadone is one of a new range of antidepressants which have similarities in action to the SSRIs but which have other specific actions on another neurotransmitter, noradrenaline, as well as serotonin. These newer drugs also act on the brain nerve cells which are activated by these neurotransmitters. Nefazadone is as effective as an antidepressant as the older tricyclic drugs and the SSRIs. Like the SSRIs, Nefazadone has less severe side effects than the tricyclics and is less toxic in overdose. Nefazadone also appears to be less likely than SSRI antidepressants to interfere with sleep.

Dosage information

Adult: 100 mg taken twice per day, which may be increased after five to seven days if necessary to 200 mg twice per day. This may be increased if necessary to **a maximum dose of 300 mg twice per day.**
Elderly and physically frail: 100-200 mg twice per day.
Children and adolescents aged 18 and under: Not recommended.

Side effects and further information

Caution is advised in patients with epilepsy or with a history of agitation or predisposition to over-excitement. Caution also advised in patients receiving electro-convulsive therapy. Side effects: Dry mouth, sleepiness, dizziness and asthenia (feelings of weakness and lack of energy). Less common side effects: Fever, chills, reduced blood pressure when standing, constipation, light-headedness, paraesthesia (pins and needles), confusion, ataxia (unsteady gait and shaky movements), amblyopia (poor eyesight) and other visual disturbance. Rarely, syncope (fainting).

　　May impair driving skills.

NEVER EXCEED THE PRESCRIBED DOSE • ALWAYS INFORM ANY DENTIST, DOCTOR OR ANAESTHETIST WHO TREATS YOU THAT YOU ARE TAKING THIS DRUG • KEEP MEDICINES OUT OF THE REACH OF CHILDREN.

PAROXETINE

Trade name	Description
Seroxat	20 mg white glossy tablets marked Seroxat 20.
	30 mg blue glossy tablets marked Seroxat 30.

General information
Paroxetine is a selective serotonin re-uptake inhibitor antidepressant. It is no more effective than older antidepressant drugs but its side effects are less severe and it is much less toxic in overdose. These factors make it preferable to tricyclic and MAOI antidepressants for most patients. The Committee on the Safety of Medicines has reported that it has received more reports of patients developing facial tics whilst on this drug than with other SSRIs and more reports of patients experiencing withdrawal effects.

Dosage information
Adult (16 and over): 20 mg per day taken as a single dose in the morning. This may be increased if necessary by increasing the dose in 10 mg steps to **a maximum dose of 50 mg per day.**
Elderly and physically frail: The maximum dose should not exceed 40 mg per day.
Children: Not recommended for the treatment of children.

Side effects and further information
Paroxetine may cause a wide variety of side effects. If a rash develops it is recommended that the drug be stopped as this could be symptomatic of vasculitis (the inflammation of small blood vessels), anaphylaxis (an allergic reaction), inflammation of the lung or fibrosis (a scarring of tissues following injury or inflammation). Nausea. Vomiting. Diarrhoea. Loss of appetite, leading to weight loss. Headache. Nervousness. Insomnia. Anxiety. Tremors. Dry mouth. Dizziness. Hypomania (elated mood, uninhibited behaviour, rapid speech and abnormal energy). Drowsiness. Convulsions. Fever. Sexual difficulties. Sweating. Less common side effects are blood changes and reduced white blood cell count. Other side effects reported are: Vaginal bleeding after withdrawal of the drug. Anaemia. Thrombocytopenia (a blood disorder which may cause bleeding into the skin, leading to bruise marks and in the event of an injury a tendency to increased bleeding). Confusion.

Use with caution in patients with liver or kidney disease, epilepsy and diabetes. Avoid in pregnancy and in breast-feeding mothers. It may impair driving ability.

NEVER EXCEED THE PRESCRIBED DOSE • ALWAYS INFORM ANY DENTIST, DOCTOR OR ANAESTHETIST WHO TREATS YOU THAT YOU ARE TAKING THIS DRUG • KEEP MEDICINES OUT OF THE REACH OF CHILDREN.

SERTRALINE

Trade name	Description
Lustral	50 mg white capsule-shaped tablets marked LTL-50. 100 mg white capsule-shaped tablets marked LTL-100.

General information

Sertraline is a selective serotonin re-uptake inhibitor antidepressant. It is no more effective than older antidepressant drugs but its side effects are less severe and it is much less toxic in overdose. These factors make it preferable to tricyclic and MAOI antidepressants for most patients.

Dosage information

Adult (16 and over): 50 mg per day, which may be increased if necessary in 50 mg steps over several weeks to **a maximum dose of 200 mg per day, which should be reduced to 50 mg per day. Doses of 150 mg per day should not be taken for more than 8 weeks.**
Elderly and physically frail: No special instructions.
Children: Not recommended for the treatment of children.

Side effects and further information

Sertraline may cause a wide variety of side effects. If a rash develops it is recommended that the drug be stopped as this could be symptomatic of vasculitis (the inflammation of small blood vessels), anaphylaxis (an allergic reaction), inflammation of the lung or fibrosis (a scarring of tissues following injury or inflammation). Nausea. Vomiting. Diarrhoea. Loss of appetite, leading to weight loss. Headache. Nervousness. Insomnia. Anxiety. Tremors. Dry mouth. Dizziness. Hypomania (elated mood, uninhibited behaviour, rapid speech and abnormal energy). Drowsiness. Convulsions. Fever. Sexual difficulties. Sweating. Less common side effects are blood changes and reduced white blood cell count. Other side effects reported are: Vaginal bleeding after withdrawal of the drug. Anaemia. Thrombocytopenia (a blood disorder which may cause bleeding into the skin, leading to bruise marks and in the event of an injury a tendency to increased bleeding). Confusion.

Use with caution in patients with liver or kidney disease, epilepsy and diabetes. Avoid in pregnancy and in breast-feeding mothers.

It may impair driving ability.

NEVER EXCEED THE PRESCRIBED DOSE • ALWAYS INFORM ANY DENTIST, DOCTOR OR ANAESTHETIST WHO TREATS YOU THAT YOU ARE TAKING THIS DRUG • KEEP MEDICINES OUT OF THE REACH OF CHILDREN.

VENLAFAXINE

Trade name	Description
Efexor	37.5 mg peach shield-shaped tablets marked Wyeth 37.5 75 mg peach shield- shaped tablets marked Wyeth 75

General information
Venlafaxine is one of a new range of antidepressants which have similarities in action to the SSRIs but which have other specific actions on another neurotransmitter, noradrenaline, as well as serotonin. These newer drugs also act on the brain nerve cells which are activated by these neurotransmitters. Venlafaxine is as effective as the older tricyclic drugs and the SSRIs. Like the SSRIs, it has less severe side effects than the tricyclics and is less toxic in overdose. May cause skin rash or allergic reaction; if this occurs seek urgent advice from your doctor.

Dosage information
Adult (16 and over): Treatment starts with 75 mg per day taken in two doses of 37.5 mg, which may be increased after several weeks if necessary to 150 mg per day in two 75 mg doses. The dose may be increased for severely depressed and hospitalised patients if necessary in steps of up to 75 mg every two to three days to a **maximum dose of 375 mg per day** and then gradually reduced.
Elderly and physically frail: No instructions.
Children and adolescents aged 18 and under: Not recommended.

Side effects and further information

Should be avoided in pregnancy and whilst breast-feeding and in patients with serious liver or kidney disease. Caution is advised in patients with a history of heart disease, epilepsy or drug dependency. Avoid abrupt withdrawal if venlafaxine has been taken for more than one week. Side effects: Dry mouth, sleepiness, dizziness and asthenia (feelings of weakness and lack of energy), sweating, nervousness, fits (if fits occur venlafaxine should be stopped), decreased sexual feelings, loss of appetite, wind. Less common side effects: Fever, chills, reduced blood pressure when standing, constipation, lightheadedness, paraesthesia (pins and needles), confusion, ataxia (unsteady gait and shaky movements), amblyopia (poor eyesight) and other visual disturbance. Rarely, syncope (fainting).

May impair driving skills.

NEVER EXCEED THE PRESCRIBED DOSE • ALWAYS INFORM ANY DENTIST, DOCTOR OR ANAESTHETIST WHO TREATS YOU THAT YOU ARE TAKING THIS DRUG • KEEP MEDICINES OUT OF THE REACH OF CHILDREN.

Other drugs used in the treatment of depression

FLUPENTHIXOL

Trade name	Description
Fluanxol	0.5 mg red tablets marked Lundbeck in black.
(see also Depixol, p. 97)	1 mg red tablets marked Lundbeck in white.

General information

Fluanxol is a low-dose preparation of flupenthixol, which is more often used to treat conditions such as schizophrenia. The use of flupenthixol in depression is a short-term, last-resort approach when all other treatments and drugs have failed. When used in low doses it is said that flupenthixol has few side effects compared with antidepressants, and it is not as dangerous in overdose. As it is used in the short-term treatment of depression at doses of approximately one-sixth of those used for schizophrenia, the side effects should be less frequent and less severe and the risk of tardive dyskinesia should be low. Flupenthixol is not recommended for severe or agitated depression or mania. The drug is claimed to exert its antidepressant action within two to three days. If no relief of the depression has been obtained after one week the drug should be withdrawn. It may impair driving ability.

Dosage information
Adult (16 and over): Treatment begins with 1 mg per day, given in one dose in the morning, which may be increased if necessary after one week to 2 mg per day. **The maximum dose for depression is 3 mg per day.** If doses of more than 2 mg per day are given, divided doses should be used, and the last dose should be given no later than 4 pm as the drug may impair sleep if taken later.
Elderly and physically frail: Treatment begins with 0.5 mg per day, given as a single dose in the morning, which may be increased if necessary to 1 mg per day. If any further increase in the dose is considered necessary, great care must be exercised. Although this is rare, **the maximum dose of 2 mg per day** may be given in divided doses of 1 mg in the morning and 1 mg at about 4 pm.
Children: Not recommended for children.

Side effects and further information
See the entry on flupenthixol, p. 98.

TRYPTOPHAN

Trade name	Description
Optimax	500 mg white capsule-shaped tablets marked OPTIMAX.

General information
Tryptophan products have been withdrawn from general use and are only available on a named patient basis for the treatment of serious depression where no other treatment or drugs are effective. Tryptophan was withdrawn from use following reports of its causing eosinophilia-myalgia (a blood condition in which certain white blood cells increase in number, with dangerous and potentially fatal consequences). It is only used to treat severe disabling depression which has not responded to other treatments for two years. Tryptophan should only be prescribed by hospital-based specialist doctors. The prescribing doctor and

the patient must be registered with the Optimax Information and Clinical Support (OPTICS) Unit. The prescriber has to complete a questionnaire after three and six months and every six months thereafter. The information collected in the questionnaires is kept under review by the Committee on the Safety of Medicines.

Dosage information
Adult (16 and over): 1 g three times per day after meals. **Maximum dose 6 g** per day.
Elderly and physically frail: The elderly and physically frail should normally receive lower doses.
Children: Not recommended for the treatment of children.

Side effects and further information
Tryptophan should be used with caution in the following conditions: Bladder disease. Nutritional deficiency, in particular of pyridoxine (vitamin B6). Tryptophan should be withdrawn if the patient suffers from headaches or blurred vision. Tryptophan interacts with other antidepressants causing excitation and confusion, with MAOI and SSRI antidepressants causing nausea and agitation.

Overdose extremely dangerous • Seek immediate medical help

PART THREE

Antipsychotic Drugs

Introduction

Antipsychotic drugs are used to control states of mind in which contact with reality is severely impaired. Such states of mind are referred to as psychotic. People in psychotic states may experience some or all of the following:

- **Hallucinations:** In which people see, hear, smell or feel touched by people or things which exist only in their minds. Amongst the most commonly reported hallucinatory experiences is the hearing of voices which may comment on the individual's behaviour, or give them instructions or be very critical of them.
- **Delusions:** Fixed irrational ideas such as the belief that your thoughts are being controlled or broadcast by some malevolent individual or power.
- **Paranoid ideas:** The belief that people are plotting or scheming against you.
- **Social withdrawal:** In which a person may withdraw from contact with people around them into themselves or into their own fantasy worlds.
- **Inappropriate emotions:** Emotions which appear to be inappropriate to the circumstances.
- **Disturbed or bizarre behaviour**.

What's in a name?
The most commonly diagnosed and best-known psychotic condition in which these drugs are used is schizophrenia which is discussed below. The same compounds are also used in low

doses to treat anxiety, nausea and vomiting. Antipsychotic drugs are amongst the most widely prescribed and important drugs in psychiatry. They are commonly referred to as 'major tranquillisers', but the term 'tranquilliser' is very misleading. Antipsychotic drugs can relieve psychotic symptoms but they do not induce anything resembling tranquillity. In fact, very often they have quite the opposite effect of causing restlessness and agitation. People taking antipsychotic drugs often find it difficult to stand or sit still. Antipsychotic drugs are also referred to as 'neuroleptics'. This term, which means a treatment which finely tunes the nerves or state of mind, is also misleading as these drugs are both powerful and have a broad range of effects beyond their useful effects. These are not predictable for any given individual, neither are they fully understood. The side effects of antipsychotic drugs are frequently severe enough to require treatment with other drugs which also have troublesome side effects. The terms tranquilliser and neuroleptic are both misnomers as they seriously understate the actual effects of these powerful drugs. For this reason this guide uses the more neutral and more accurate term 'antipsychotic' to describe them.

The first of the antipsychotics, chlorpromazine, was derived from a substance called phenothiazine which was discovered in 1883. Phenothiazine was used in the mid-1930s as an insecticide, a treatment for parasitic worms and as an antiseptic for bladder infections. Chlorpromazine was first used in surgery to improve the effects of anaesthetics. In 1952 French researchers described how chlorpromazine produced an effect which they described as 'artificial hibernation'. They noted that whilst patients who were administered chlorpromazine did not lose consciousness, they did have a tendency to become sleepy and show a marked lack of interest in what was going on around them. The value of this sense of detachment from events prior to surgery is easily understood. The first trials of chlorpromazine for psychiatry showed it to be effective in reducing psychotic symptoms in patients diagnosed as agitated schizophrenics. It was the first drug in psychiatry whose effects were specific to psychotic symptoms. Previously the drugs that were used tended simply to sedate them heavily. Chlorpromazine transformed the face of psychiatry.

Before the advent of chlorpromazine, mental hospitals provided little more than custodial care combined with heavy sedation. A booklet produced for doctors by a leading manufacturer of antipsychotic drugs makes the following observation: 'People with experience in psychiatric care agree that the introduction of chlorpromazine in psychiatric hospitals has reduced the time patients spend in seclusion and restraint'. This is true but it avoids the issue that drugs like chlorpromazine may be used as an alternative and insidious method of restraint. A form of restraint which may look less alarming to the onlooker than a straight jacket but which may be experienced by the restrained individual as much more distressing. The terms 'chemical cosh' and 'liquid-straight jacket' refer to a reality in which antipsychotic drugs may be used to control people's behaviour rather than the symptoms of mental illness.

Antipsychotic drugs have improved the quality of life for many hundreds of thousands of seriously distressed people. But they are not universally effective and they are far from being trouble free. Antipsychotics, particularly when they are prescribed in high doses, can have a wide range of life-diminishing side effects and present serious long-term hazards to the patient. The benefits of these powerful drugs are frequently overstated whilst their side effects and hazards often tend to be overlooked or minimised. In a climate of public panic about the failures of care in the community, drugs are often seen to provide an easy solution to complex and barely understood problems.

Some people believe that the introduction of chlorpromazine and its chemical cousins led directly to the reduction of the numbers of people confined in mental hospitals. However, a more careful reading of history shows that the decline in the number of psychiatric in-patients began soon after the end of World War II, some ten years before the introduction of chlorpromazine into psychiatric practice. However, chlorpromazine as the first symptom-specific drug did add to the impetus to the movement towards care in the community.

Chlorpromazine (trade name Largactil) remains one of the most widely prescribed antipsychotic drugs in Britain. Since it was first used in psychiatry many similar drugs have been introduced. Some critics believe that there are now far too many similar compounds available. They argue that rational prescribing is made more difficult by the plethora of 'me too' drugs competing for the attention and loyalties of prescribers. There are few significant differences in the antipsychotic properties of many of these drugs, although some have different side-effect profiles.

Some are more sedating whilst others may have more stimulant effects. The choice as to which drug should be prescribed to a particular patient will often depend more on its side effects than on its effectiveness in relieving psychotic symptoms. Chlorpromazine as the first of the antipsychotics is the one against which the effects of the others are compared for reference.

Antipsychotic drugs may be taken by mouth in tablet form or as a syrup, or by injection. Depot antipsychotics such as fluphenazine (Modecate) and flupenthixol (Depixol) are administered by injection and their effects can last for several weeks. They may be administered at intervals of between one and four weeks (people who need to observe religious dietary laws may wish to know that the active drug is suspended in sesame oil). The advantage of depot drugs is that patients do not have to remember to take pills regularly. In ideal circumstances, once the appropriate dose of a depot antipsychotic drug has been established no other similar drug should be necessary. However, many patients regularly receive two or more similar antipsychotic drugs in the same course of treatment, which can expose them to increased side effects and a higher risk of suffering permanent damage to their nervous systems. The practice of prescribing two or more similar drugs concurrently is referred to as 'poly-pharmacy'. Poly-pharmacy is justified by some prescribers who argue that it allows for the fine tuning of doses for individual patients. However, numerous specialist researchers have expressed serious concern about the prevalence of poly-pharmacy in psychiatry.

Antipsychotic drugs are not helpful for everyone and neither do they always prevent people who take them regularly from suffering relapses. An English study (Leff and Wing, 1971)[1] which looked at a very large number of people diagnosed as schizophrenic revealed that seven in one hundred did not have any positive response to antipsychotic drugs and that twenty-four out of a hundred relapsed within a year of taking them. American research (Cole, Goldberg and Klerman, 1964)[2] shows that one patient in twenty failed to show any positive response and that between one in ten and one in five relapsed whilst taking the

[1] Leff, J. P. and Wing, J. K.: 'Trial of Maintenance Therapy in Schizophrenia, *British Medical Journal*, 5, pp.559-604, 1971.
[2] Cole, J. O., Goldberg S. C. and Klerman, G. L.: 'Phenothiazine Treatment in Acute Schizophrenia', *Archives of General Psychiatry*, 10, pp.246-61, 1964.

medication within the first six months of treatment. Recent research (Crow et al., 1986)[3] which compared the progress of people who after their first episode of schizophrenia took a 'placebo' with those who took a real antipsychotic drug found that within two years 58 per cent of those taking the real drug had relapsed whilst 78 per cent of those receiving the placebo had relapsed. Findings like these show that most patients are likely to benefit for most of the time from taking antipsychotic medication. But they do not support the enthusiasm with which these drugs are advocated or prescribed – often two or more concurrently and frequently in very high doses. Neither do such findings support the view that extending the legal powers of psychiatrists to administer these drugs forcibly in the community is either just or likely to be effective.

People respond differently to antipsychotic drugs. Some are more prone to experiencing severe side effects and there is no formula for establishing the dose required to achieve a maximum control of symptoms with a minimum of side effects. In ideal circumstances when an antipsychotic drug is first prescribed the dose should be as low as possible and be increased as necessary to achieve the maximum benefit for the distressed person. Dose levels should also be regularly reviewed but often people are routinely prescribed high doses which are seldom, if ever, reviewed. Some people genuinely do require higher doses than others but often it appears that services are geared toward organisational uniformity and convenience rather than the specific needs of individual patients. Generally speaking, the higher the prescribed dose, the more likely it is that the side effects will be severe. Some patients simply do not respond to treatment with antipsychotic drugs. Such patients are those at most risk of being given mega-doses in the futile hope that that some benefit may be achieved. Such patients are exposed to more severe side effects and an increased risk of neurological damage.

Research into psychiatric prescribing practices (Johnson and Wright, 1990)[4] reviewed the evidence as to whether very high doses of antipsychotics may be more effective for patients who do not benefit from standard doses. They concluded that 'The

---

[3] Crow, T. J., Macmillan, J. S., Johnson, A. L. and Johnson, E. C.: 'The Northwick Park Study of First Episodes of Schizophrenia; A Controlled Study of Neuroleptic Treatment'; *British Journal of Psychiatry*, 148, pp. 120–7. 1986.

consensus view is that very high doses have not proved benefi-cial'. In the same paper the authors cited a number of reports which showed that very high doses of antipsychotic drugs made some patient's symptoms worse. In the light of a great deal of research which has failed to show any substantial benefits from using very high doses it is difficult to understand why they are so often prescribed in this way. Whatever the reasons, it is a matter for concern not only because of the harm such prescribing does to patients, but also because it risks discrediting potentially help-ful treatment in the eyes of people who could benefit from it. A hospital ward or local day centre full of over-medicated patients does not inspire confidence.

Under the provisions of the 1983 Mental Health Act drugs may be administered without the consent of patients (for details of consent procedures under the MHA, 1983 (see p. 151). There are circumstances in which it may be necessary for the safety and well-being of a mentally distressed person, or for the safety of others, that drugs should be administered without the patient's consent. Even when such powers are not present patients may be pressured to take the drugs. These factors of compulsion and pressure place heavy moral obligations on those responsible for administering treatment. They have an obligation to be as sure as possible that the drug's benefits significantly outweigh its adverse effects and any risks of the treatment to the patient's safety. This demands an awareness and sensitivity to the patient's experi-ences of the drug's effects.

Getting the most from antipsychotic drugs
In conditions like schizophrenia it is usually necessary for the patient to continue taking antipsychotic drugs over long periods of time. For some people it may mean taking the drugs for the rest of their lives. It is usually best to start with the lowest dose necessary to achieve the best relief of symptoms with the mini-mum of discomfort to the patient. As it is not possible to predict how these drugs will affect the individual patient, finding the

[4] Johnson, D.A.W. and Wright, N.F., 'Drug Prescribing to Chronic Hospital In-Patients on Depot Injections. Repeat Surveys over 18 years,' *British Journal of Psychiatry*, 56, pp. 827–34. 1990.

See also a review of literature on psychiatric prescribing in Rogers, A., Pil-grim, D. and Lacey, R. in 'Experiencing Psychiatry User views of Services.' (Macmillan) pp.121–61. 1993.

correct dose inevitably involves trial and error. It is recommended that the drug is started at the lowest end of its dosage
range and gradually increased until the appropriate dose for the
individual patient has been established. Many people will experience the common side effects of these drugs very early on in
their treatment, and if these are troublesome another drug may
be prescribed to counter them (for details of medications for side
effects, see p.132–135). Some psychiatrists routinely prescribe
medication for side effects at the same time as they prescribe an
antipsychotic, but this practice is criticised by the World Health
Organisation. Medications for side effects may reduce the effectiveness of antipsychotic drugs whilst increasing their hazards.
Patients are likely to get the most benefit from antipsychotic
medication when it is prescribed at the lowest effective dose and
with as few other drugs as possible. Once an individual's symptoms have been controlled it is often possible to reduce the dose
of the drug to fine tune the balance between symptom control
and side effects.

Some patients may forget to take their pills regularly whilst
others may unwisely stop taking them. There are patients who
may develop a fixed belief that the drugs are poisoning them
(although such a belief may not in itself be sufficient reason to
force treatment on a patient). For these reasons patients should
be given 'depot' injections of drugs which last for weeks at a
time. These patients may receive monthly injections in their own
homes from a community psychiatric nurse or in a special clinic.
Many patients in hospitals receive monthly depot injections. It is
doubtful that there is any advantage to the patient in combining
depot with other antipsychotic compounds over extended periods of time, although in the short term such combinations may
help to establish the optimum dose for the individual. Some
people are concerned that depot injections may be used more for
the convenience of doctors and nurses than for the benefit of
their patients. Concern has been voiced that so-called 'depot
clinics' operate more like production lines than treatment services tailored to the needs of individuals.

Many patients are prescribed antidepressants with antipsychotic drugs. Some antipsychotic drugs can cause patients to feel
depressed and some people who suffer from schizophrenia may
feel depressed. However, the combination of antipsychotic and
antidepressant medications is controversial. In reviewing the

studies of such combination prescribing, Johnson and Wright (1990)[5] conclude, 'It is clear that at the present time the prescription of antidepressants (concurrently with antipsychotics) must be regarded as a therapeutic trial. Since there are possible risks of schizophrenic deterioration these patients must receive careful supervision.'

There is a growing amount of evidence that antipsychotic drugs are a great deal more effective when given as part of a comprehensive treatment plan which includes help with the daily problems of living. Social and emotional stress are the most clearly identifiable factors in causing relapse in schizophrenia. Serious mental illness and distress cause a great deal of anguish and stress to those closest to the sufferer. If these stresses are not dealt with, the chances of the patient experiencing a serious relapse are considerably increased. The families of mentally ill people often need help and understanding in order to cope with the strains imposed on them. Research shows that when such help is given that it can be very effective in preventing relapses.

There is an increasing number of studies which show that patients who receive social support as well as drugs do dramatically better than patients who receive drugs only. Two studies are worthy of mention. In the first (Leff et al., 1982[6], and also referred to in a 1989 study by Falloon[7] et al.,) the progress of two groups of people diagnosed as schizophrenic was monitored over two years. One group received antipsychotic drugs only, whilst the other received social and family support as well as antipsychotic drugs. After two years, more than three-quarters of those who received only the drug had suffered a serious relapse, whilst only one-fifth of those who had received the drug and family support had relapsed. In the second similar study the comparative relapse rates between the two groups over a two-

[5] Johnson, D. A. W. and Wright, N. F.: op. cit., p. 830.
[6] Leff, J., Kuipers, L. and Berkowitz, R.: 'A Trial of Social Intervention in the Families of Schizophrenic Patients', *British Journal of Psychiatry*, 141, pp. 121–34, 1982.
[7] Falloon, 1. R. H., Boyd, J. L., McGill, C. W., Razani, J., Moss, H. B. and Gilderman, A. M.: 'Family Management in the Prevention of Exacerbation of Schizophrenia: A Controlled Study, *New England Journal of Medicine*, 306, p.1437, 1989.

See also Berkowitz, R., Shavit, N. et al,: 'A Trial of Family Therapy Versus a Relatives Group for Schizophrenia', *British Journal of Psychiatry*, 154, pp. 58–66, 1989.

year period was equally startling. Eighty-three per cent of those on drugs alone relapsed within two years whilst only 17 per cent of those who had received drugs and family support had relapsed. It is a matter of sadness that the encouraging findings of research studies such as these have not been translated into action on a more widespread basis. Despite the rhetoric of community care too few hospitals or community teams seem to have the inclination or resources to co-ordinate the medical and social aspects of care properly. For a disturbing number of patients the drugs-only regime is all that is on offer. Apart from preventing unnecessary distress to patients and their relatives, approaches such as those outlined above may save money by reducing the need for people to be admitted to hospital.

Schizophrenia

Before describing the drugs used to treat serious mental illnesses, it is worth taking a closer look at the particular illness they are most used for.

Schizophrenia is a serious mental illness in which a group of experiences appear together in one person. Briefly, these symptoms or experiences are: hallucinations (sensory experiences for which no external cause exists, such as hearing voices or feeling things that are not there); delusions (irrational beliefs, such as the belief that one's thoughts are being controlled or broadcast); markedly illogical thought processes; inappropriate emotional responses; social withdrawal; blunted emotions and grossly disturbed behaviour. In the industrialised world schizophrenia is said to affect approximately one out of two hundred people. The symptoms of schizophrenia place heavy burdens on the lives of its sufferers, and the prejudices they encounter in their communities add substantially to those burdens. Nobody really knows what causes schizophrenia but research into the structure and activity of the brain, as well as into genetics, sociology and psychology, has brought promising pointers to some of its possible causes.

The experience of schizophrenia has been compared to the experience of a dream or nightmare. In a dream our minds are flooded by a jumble of thoughts and emotions which do not conform to any logical patterns; we are pitched into a world of vivid imagery in which the familiar and the strange are woven together. We may be terrified by threatening and bizarre images, sounds and feelings, or haunted by unseen menaces. We may feel ourselves to be masters of all around us, with unlimited powers to control people and events. We may hear other people's thoughts, walk on or under water, fly, or go skateboarding with the Queen Mother. We may believe ourselves to be controlled by menacing, unseen forces. Our emotions might be entirely inappropriate to the events in our dream. We might laugh at the death of a loved one or feel downcast at a moment of triumph. Our dreams seldom unfold with the neat and ordered story-lines of films. In dreams the chaotic and the fantastical are as real to us as the events around us in our everyday lives. Such dream states resemble the experience of schizophrenia. When they are experienced during a person's waking hours, they are described as 'psychotic', meaning that they come from within the psyche rather than from external reality. Psychotic states are distinguished from the neurotic by the fact that they involve a break with reality. In a neurotic state the individual has irrational fears or anxieties but remains in contact with and accessible to events and people around him.

Even in our waking moments we may glimpse the experience of schizophrenia. How many of us are half-convinced that we can make it rain by washing the car or going out without a raincoat? This is not so far removed from a paranoid delusion.

The foundations of the modern concept of schizophrenia were laid during the latter part of the nineteenth century by Emil Kraepelin, one of the pioneers of modern psychiatry. He described and classified the group of symptoms as *dementia praecox,* the dementia of early life, but it was the Swiss psychiatrist Eugene Bleuler who used the term schizophrenia to denote the concept of a split mind. Kraepelin and Bleuler pioneered modern diagnostic conventions regarding schizophrenia.

Research into the possibility that abnormal brain chemistry is a primary cause of schizophrenia has been pursued with vigour and enthusiasm for over a century. However, so far there have been more unfulfilled promises of imminent breakthroughs than hard knowledge. With the use of brain scans, more recent research has identified evidence of small areas of brain atrophy in some but not all people diagnosed as schizophrenic. Although roughly a quarter of such patients have these abnormalities, similar abnormalities are seen in many people who do not suffer from schizophrenia. Another line of research has been to measure the responses of people with schizophrenia and their relatives to a variety of stimuli, such as flashing lights and noises. This research indicates that sufferers from schizophrenia, along with some of their relatives, have abnormally high responses to these stimuli. These findings suggest that schizophrenia arises from the way in which the brain processes information.

Geneticists, on the other hand, have been searching for an abnormal or delinquent gene as a factor in causing schizophrenia, but not all research in this field has been rigorous in gathering and interpreting its data. Franz Kallmann, once regarded as the leading pioneer of genetic research into schizophrenia, published a series of findings from studies of twins purporting to show an overwhelming statistical link between heredity and schizophrenia. But Kallmann, who was a leading light in the eugenics movement in pre-war Germany before he emigrated to the USA, was discovered to have fiddled his results. Kallmann's name continues to appear in learned articles and psychiatric textbooks, despite the fact that his work has been systematically discredited by numerous scholarly reviewers. More recent and more rigorous studies into twins have shown that heredity may be a predisposing factor in schizophrenia. But critics of this research argue that environmental factors may have more significance to this apparent increased susceptibility to mental illness.

On the socio-economic front there are some facts about the distribution of schizophrenia which seem relevant. Sociological research shows that schizophrenia is much more commonly diagnosed amongst economically disadvantaged populations than others. Social factors have also been shown to be significant to the rate of relapse amongst schizophrenia sufferers. The possibility that disturbed or confusing relationships within families may cause schizophrenia has also been suggested. Subsequent research and observation, however, has neither confirmed nor lent credibility to this theory. The concept of the 'schizogenic family' (that is, a family which causes a member to become schizophrenic) has not been helpful to sufferers or their families. It has left a legacy of blame for families. The ways in which sufferers from schizophrenia and their families interact can affect the rate at which relapses occur, and help given to those families can reduce the relapse rate. As I have shown above, a number of studies have shown not only that drugs work more effectively when given along with support to the families, but also that drugs may be given in lower doses with equal effectiveness when such support is given.

The present state of understanding is that schizophrenia is a multicausal collection of illnesses, but none of the evidence is absolutely conclusive. As much as we might wish it to be otherwise, for the foreseeable future the treatment of schizophrenia will continue to be focused on the use of imperfect antipsychotic drugs. The formidable financial might of the pharmaceutical industry sets most of the research agendas in mental health. Some argue that this bias blights research into social and psychological factors in the causation and treatments for schizophrenia. Like it or not, the everyday reality for most schizophrenia sufferers is that the main focus in their treatment centres around the use of antipsychotic drugs. In these circumstances the real issue to be addressed is how we make the best use of these drugs. This means that the context in which they used must be given as much attention as their effects.

So far the debate over the merits of care in the community has been uninformed by an understanding of the actual, rather than the assumed, effectiveness of antipsychotic drugs.

Whatever its causes, mental illness occurs within a social context and has social consequences. Social factors play a major part in causing people to relapse whether they are taking drugs or not. Drugs have an important part to play in helping those of us who suffer to recover from mental illness and distress. Mental hospitals often seem to be universities of helplessness presided over by professors of applied passivity. Too often these old institutional traditions are being carried over into the community. If care in the community is to work, the patient needs to be recruited into the multi-disciplinary team as an active participant in his own recovery. This will involve coming clean with people about the realities of medication and helping people to understand its relevance to them and how they get the best from it. It is simply not good enough to ignore or dismiss people's experience of side effects or their legitimate concerns about the long-term consequences of treatment. With the honourable exception of the work of a few multidisciplinary teams, the treatment of schizophrenia in Britain is limited to the use of drugs to control its symptoms.

Writing the prescription is the easy part of treating mental illness. The difficult part usually starts after the diagnosis and treatment, when the mentally ill person has to find or learn ways of getting by on a pittance in the community – a community which at best may be indifferent and at worst downright hostile. To do this requires access to a much more complex range of skills than those required to be a compliant patient. The acid test of the quality of mental health services is not how scientifically learned the staff are, but how acceptable the treatment they give would be to the man or woman in the street. By this test, many services fall very far short of the ideal. The prospect of madness is frightening but so is the prospect of becoming a psychiatric patient. Very few patients can be identified by the strange and often terrifying experiences of their inner worlds. What identifies patients to most strangers is not their madness but the side effects of their medication. This is not a call to ban or even to reduce the use of these drugs; it is a plea that they should be used with the utmost care and sensitivity. In an increasingly competitive market economy in which the 'mentally ill' are seen as a menacing burden, the spectre of community care out of a syringe looms menacingly.

Six-point guide to getting the most from antipsychotic drugs

In order to maximise the benefits and minimise the side effects of antipsychotic drugs the following points should be borne in mind:

1. Antipsychotic drugs should be used at the lowest possible dose which achieves the maximum relief of symptoms and the minimum of adverse effects.
2. Prescriptions should be as simple as possible. Once the optimum dosage level has been established for the individual, no more than one antipsychotic drug should be routinely prescribed at any one time.
3. If medication to control side effects is necessary its use should be regularly reviewed and stopped as soon as possible.
4. Antipsychotic drugs should not be prescribed in combination with other psychiatric drugs unless there are compelling reasons to do so. Such combination prescribing should be sub-

ject to close and regular review and should be stopped as soon as possible.

5. Antipsychotic drugs should be used as a part of a comprehensive treatment plan which includes help to reduce life stresses for the patient. Families and carers should also receive help and support in order to diminish the stresses they experience and thus to protect the well-being of the patient.

6. People receiving treatment with antipsychotic drugs should be cautious in their use of alcohol.

FAST FACTS ABOUT ANTIPSYCHOTIC DRUGS

Purpose

The treatment of schizophrenia and other conditions where psychotic symptoms are present. The short term control of agitation, dangerous behaviour and mania. In very low doses, and over short periods of time, the treatment of severe anxiety.

How do I take the drug?

In tablet form or by injection or drunk as a syrup. People may receive antipsychotic drugs in all these forms concurrently but this is rarely justified in the long term.

When do I take it?

In tablet or syrup form, as directed by the prescribing doctor. Injections may be given in emergencies. With the long-acting or depot preparations, it may be given on a monthly basis.

How long does it take to work?

These drugs affect people differently and will act more rapidly for some than for others. The time a drug takes to work will vary, depending on the particular compound used, the dose and on the method of administration. When administered by injection some of the drug's actions will occur very rapidly. When the drug is first taken it may take up to three weeks before it begins to act on symptoms.

Should I expect to experience side effects?

Yes, but some of these may be more severe when you first begin to take the drug.

What are the most common side effects?

Agitation, restlessness, drowsiness, apathy, nightmares, depression, nasal congestion, trembling hands, blurred vision, sensitivity to sunlight (a risk of sunburn), impotence, reduced capacity for orgasm, changes in menstrual cycle, weight gain, reduced body temperature, reduced blood pressure.

continued

Parkinsonism. With long-term use tardive dyskinesia and drug-induced psychosis. (see pp. 129–130). NB Some of the side effects vary in severity between different compounds. For fuller details consult the individual drugs listing.

What should I do if I experience other distressing side effects?

You should always inform your doctor about side effects as it may be possible to reduce their severity by a reduction in dose or by drugs prescribed specifically to reduce these effects (see p. 125).

How long should I continue to take it?

It may be necessary for you to continue taking this drug for years. This will depend on your condition and individual needs. You should review the dose you take and the need to continue with the drug at least every six months with the prescribing doctor.

Is it addictive?

No, but you may develop a physical dependency on the drug which may cause you to experience muscular discomfort and insomnia if you suddenly stop taking the drug. You will not develop any craving for the drug, nor will you need to increase the dose to gain its benefits.

Antipsychotic drugs are often prescribed with other medications to counter their side effects. These drugs are listed and described on p. 131.

ANTIPSYCHOTIC DRUGS ARE PRESCRIBED FOR SERIOUS MENTAL ILLNESS OR DISTRESS • IT IS INADVISABLE AND POTENTIALLY HAZARDOUS TO STOP TAKING THEM AGAINST MEDICAL ADVICE AS YOU MAY EXPERIENCE A SERIOUS RECURRENCE OF THE CONDITION FOR WHICH THE DRUG WAS PRESCRIBED • IF YOU ARE WORRIED ABOUT THE EFFECTS OF THE DRUG ALWAYS CONSULT YOUR DOCTOR • IF YOU ARE UNABLE TO RESOLVE THE PROBLEM WITH YOUR OWN DOCTOR YOU SHOULD SEEK A SECOND MEDICAL OPINION

BENPERIDOL

Trade name	Description
Anquil	250 microgram white tablets marked JANSSEN on one side and 0.25 on the other.

General information
An antipsychotic drug whose manufacturers claim is useful in the control of deviant and antisocial sexual behaviour. It has been advertised for its ability to suppress masturbation in people with learning difficulties. A very controversial drug whose value according to the British National Formulary 'is not established'.

Dosage information
Adult (16 and over): Between 0.25–1.5 mg daily in divided doses.
Elderly and physically frail: Treatment begins with half the adult dose.
Children: Not recommended for children.

Side effects and further information
If benperidol has any place in the treatment of mental illness it is a very limited one. It is not as sedating as chlorpromazine but it causes inner agitation, physical restlessness, a mask-like facial appearance, tremors, and muscular rigidity more frequently.

CHLORPROMAZINE

Trade name	Description
Largactil	10 mg, 25 mg, 50 mg and 100 mg off-white coated tablets. Clear golden-brown syrup containing 25 mg per 5 ml. Orange suspension to be diluted with water containing 100 mg per 5 ml. Ampoules of pale straw-coloured liquid for injection.
Under generic name	10 mg, 25 mg, 50 mg and 100 mg white coated tablets. Elixir (liquid) containing 25 mg per 5 ml. Ampoules for injection. 100 mg suppositories for insertion into rectum.

General information

Chlorpromazine was the first effective antipsychotic drug to be used in psychiatry and remains one of the most widely prescribed drugs in this group. It is the drug against which all the other antipsychotics are compared in order to measure their effectiveness and side effects. Chlorpromazine is an effective treatment for symptoms such as hallucinations, thought disorders and delusions caused by schizophrenia and other psychotic conditions. It may also be used to control violent and difficult behaviour. In common with other antipsychotic compounds it is impossible to predict the dose of chlorpromazine an individual patient will need for the relief of symptoms. The dose level needs to be established through trial and error and by gradually increasing it until the desired effect has been achieved. It is often possible to reduce the dose once the patient's condition has been stabilised.

Chlorpromazine is an effective antipsychotic medicine but patients may suffer a relapse whilst taking it. There is also a small number of patients who do not benefit from antipsychotic drugs and some whose condition will worsen if they take them. It is not possible to predict which patients will not benefit from antipsychotic drugs, neither is it possible to predict which patients will suffer a relapse whilst taking these drugs.

Dosage information

Adult (16 and over): For the control of schizophrenia and other psychoses, serious agitation, over-excitement or violent and dangerous behaviour. *By mouth:* treatment begins with 25 mg three times per day or a single dose of 75 mg at night. This dose may be increased according to the response of the patient to a normal maintenance dose of between 75 mg and 300 mg per day. Occasionally, in the case of severe symptoms, the daily dose may be increased to **a maximum of 1000 mg per day**. Doses which exceed this are controversial.

Dose by deep intramuscular injection: For the relief of very severe symptoms. 25–50 mg every six to eight hours.

Dose by rectum: 100 mg suppositories every six to eight hours.

Elderly and physically frail: One-third to a half of the normal adult dose. Elderly people are more prone to side effects and to suffering from tardive dyskinesia (see pp. 129–130).

Children: Between the ages of one to five, 500 micrograms per kilo of the child's body weight. Between the ages of six and twelve, one-third to half the adult dose. The use of antipsychotic drugs for children is controversial.

Side effects and further information
Chlorpromazine causes more sedation and drowsiness than other antipsychotic compounds (see p. 125 for a full description of side effects).

Prolonged use may cause tardive dyskinesia, a condition which causes people to develop facial tics and other involuntary movements (for a fuller description of tardive dyskinesia and its side effects, see pp. 129–130).

Caution is advised in handling liquid forms of chlorpromazine as it can cause unpleasant skin reactions.

CLOZAPINE

Trade name	Description
Clozaril	25 mg yellow scored tablets. 100 mg yellow scored tablets (for use in hospitals only).

General information
Because of the high incidence of agranulocytosis in patients treated with clozapine it is usually only prescribed when a patient cannot tolerate, or his or her symptoms are not relieved by, another antipsychotic drug. Agranulocytosis is a serious and potentially fatal blood disorder which causes damage to the bone marrow. For this reason clozapine's use is restricted to prescribers, pharmacists and patients registered with the Clozaril Patient Monitoring Group. Before clozapine is used the patient's blood must be tested for any existing disorder. During the first 18 weeks of treatment the patient's blood should be tested every week to monitor any changes caused by the drug. Thereafter a blood test is necessary every two weeks. If any signs of blood disorder occur the drug should be withdrawn. Patients who have remained stable on clozapine for 12 months or more may only require blood tests every four weeks.

Clozapine should be used with extreme caution in patients with infections, liver or kidney disorders, epilepsy, heart disease, enlarged prostate gland, glaucoma (a condition in which there is abnormal pressure in the eye) and paralytic ileus (an obstruction in the intestines).

Dosage information

Adult (16 and over): Treatment begins with 25–50 mg per day which may be increased or decreased according to the response of the patient. If a larger dose is necessary this should be done by increasing the dose by 25–50 mg per day (for elderly people, by 25 mg) over a period of seven to fourteen days, to reach 300 mg per day). The drug may be taken as a single dose at bedtime. The usual dose for psychotic symptoms is between 200–450 mg per day. **The maximum dose is 900 mg per day** which should be reduced to a usual maintenance dose of between 150–300 mg per day.

Children: Clozapine should not be used to treat children.

Side effects and further information

Clozapine may cause potentially fatal blood disorders, the symptoms of which are fever and ulceration of the mouth and throat which may rapidly lead to collapse and death. Clozapine should be avoided by people with a history of drug-caused blood disorders, bone marrow disorders and epilepsy. It should be avoided in people who have become psychotic as a result of drug or alcohol abuse, coma and depression.

Clozapine should not be taken during pregnancy or whilst breast-feeding. The side effects of clozapine include: Excessive salivation. Dry mouth. Reduced blood pressure which may cause patients to feel faint when they stand. Physical and psychological restlessness. Increased body temperature. Tremors. Inner feelings of agitation. Drowsiness. Blurred vision. Muscular rigidity and a mask-like facial appearance. An increase in the risk of suffering epileptic fits.

Rare side effects include: Arrhythmia (changes in the heart rate, palpitations, breathlessness and chest pains). Delirium. Liver disease. Neuroleptic malignant syndrome (a rare and potentially fatal condition caused by antipsychotic drugs, the symptoms of which are an increase in body temperature, sweating, jerky involuntary movements of the limbs, drowsiness, rapid breathing, stupor, and coma).

DROPERIDOL

Trade name	Description
Droleptan	10 mg yellow tablets marked JANSSEN on one side and D over 10 on the other. Clear liquid to be taken orally. Ampoules for injection.

General information

Droperidol is used to boost the effects of pain-relieving drugs in surgery as a pre-medication and as a treatment for post-operative nausea. It is also used to treat the side effects of nausea and vomiting caused by drugs used in the treatment of cancer. In psychiatry it is used to calm agitated, manic and psychotic patients. Its effects are identical to those of haloperidol. In this guide only information about droperidol's use in psychiatry is given.

Dosage information

Adult (16 and over): For sedation and emergency control of mania. *By mouth:* 5–10 mg repeated every four to six hours as necessary. **Maximum dose: 15 mg every four hours.**
By injection: up to 10 mg repeated every four to six hours as necessary.
Elderly and physically frail: Treatment begins with half the adult dose.
Children: 0.5–1 mg per day, which if necessary should be increased with care. The use of antipsychotic drugs in children is controversial and should be avoided if possible.

Side effects and further information

Droperidol is less sedating than chlorpromazine but more often causes inner agitation, physical restlessness, a mask-like facial appearance, tremors and muscular rigidity. Prolonged use may cause tardive dyskinesia, a condition which causes facial tics and other involuntary movements (for a fuller description of tardive dyskinesia, see pp. 129–130).

FLUPENTHIXOL

Trade name	Description
Depixol	3 mg yellow tablets printed with Lundbeck on one side. Straw-coloured liquid in ampoule, vial or syringe for injection.

General information

Flupenthixol is a potent and rapidly acting antipsychotic which may be administered by daily doses or given as an injection which will last for between two and four weeks (see flupenthixol decanoate, p. 118). When given as a daily treatment it is relatively short-acting. It is said to have an alerting effect on withdrawn patients, which may be related to the feelings of restlessness which are a common side effect of this particular group of antipsychotic drugs.

Dosage information

Adult (16 and over): Treatment begins with 3–9 mg twice daily, increased or decreased according to the response of the patient. **The maximum dose is 18 mg (six 3 mg tablets) per day.**
Elderly and physically frail: Should be avoided for the treatment of elderly, confused or senile people.
Children: The manufacturers recommend that flupenthixol should not be used to treat children.

Side effects and further information

In approximately 25 per cent of patients flupenthixol causes extrapyramidal side effects: inner agitation, physical restlessness, a mask-like facial appearance, tremors and muscular rigidity. Prolonged use may cause tardive dyskinesia, a condition which causes facial tics and other involuntary movements (for a fuller description of tardive dyskinesia and its effects, see p. 129).

FLUPHENAZINE HYDROCHLORIDE

Trade name	Description
Moditen	1 mg pink tablets. 2.5 mg yellow tablets. 5 mg white tablets.

General information

Fluphenazine is a potent antipsychotic drug used to control the symptoms of schizophrenia, extreme agitation, withdrawal, dangerous behaviour and mania. It is said to be particularly useful in treating paranoid psychosis. It may be given as a daily dose or as a depot injection lasting from ten days to three weeks (see fluphenazine decanoate, p. 120). It is more likely to cause extrapyramidal side effects (see below) than some other antipsychotic compounds.

Dosage information

Adult (16 and over): For anxiety and non-psychotic behaviour disturbances: 1 mg twice daily, increased if necessary to 2 mg twice daily.

For schizophrenia, psychotic withdrawal, mania and paranoid psychosis: Treatment begins with between 2.5–10 mg per day in two or three doses, depending on the severity of the symptoms. The dose may be increased or decreased according to the response of the patient. **The maximum dose is 20 mg per day.** Higher doses should only be given with great caution.

Elderly and physically frail: As elderly people are more likely to suffer from side effects they should be treated with lower doses. Doses above 10 mg per day should only be used with great caution in elderly people.

Children: The manufacturers recommend that fluphenazine should not be used to treat children.

Side effects and further information

Fluphenazine should be avoided in comatose patients and patients who suffer from diseased blood vessels in the brain; phaeochromocytoma (a tumour in the adrenal gland which causes increased blood pressure and heart rate, palpitations and headaches), liver disease, kidney disease, heart disease, or severe depression.

Fluphenazine is less sedating than chlorpromazine but it is more likely to cause extrapyramidal side effects (inner agitation, physical restlessness, a mask-like facial appearance, tremors and muscular rigidity). Prolonged use may cause tardive dyskinesia, a condition which causes facial tics and other involuntary movements for a fuller description of tardive dyskinesia see pp. 129–130).

HALOPERIDOL

Trade name	Description
Dozic	Liquid to be taken by mouth containing 1 mg per ml.
Haldol	5 mg blue tablets.
	10 mg yellow tablets.
	Liquid to be taken by mouth containing 2 mg per ml.
Serenace	0.5 mg green capsules.
	1.6 mg pink tablets.
	10 mg pale pink tablets.
	20 mg dark pink tablets.
	Liquid to be taken by mouth containing 2 mg per ml.
	Ampoules for injection.

General information

Haloperidol is a highly potent antipsychotic which can act rapidly to control the symptoms of schizophrenia, mania and dangerous behaviour. It is less sedating than chlorpromazine but its other side effects may be more severe and more frequent. In particular, the side effects which give the patient a zombie-like appearance and cause physical and psychological restlessness and depression are more common.

Dosage information

Adult (16 and over): For the control of the symptoms of schizophrenia, mania, extreme agitation and dangerous behaviour. *By mouth:* Treatment begins with between 1.5–20 mg per day in divided doses, gradually increased or decreased according to the response of the patient. **The maximum dose is 100 mg, occasionally 200 mg per day** in very disturbed patients. *By injection:* 2–10 mg, increasing to 30 mg for emergency control, then repeated injections of 5 mg every four to eight hours. In extreme circumstances the injections may be given hourly until control of the symptoms has been achieved.

Elderly and physically frail: Half the adult starting dose, to a **maximum dose of 4 mg per day.**

Children: *By mouth:* 25–50 micrograms per kilogram of body weight daily, to a **maximum dose of 10 mg daily;** or for adolescents (13–16) up to a **maximum dose of 30 mg (in exceptional circumstances up to 60 mg per day may be given**). The administration of haloperidol by injection to children is *not* recommended. The use of antipsychotic drugs to treat children is controversial.

Side effects and further information
Haloperidol is less sedating than chlorpromazine but is more likely to cause extrapyramidal side effects (inner agitation, physical restlessness, a mask-like facial appearance, tremors and muscular rigidity). Prolonged use may cause tardive dyskinesia, a condition which causes facial tics and other involuntary movements (for a fuller description of tardive dyskinesia see pp. 129–130).

LOXAPINE

Trade name	Description
Loxapac	10 mg yellow and green capsules.
	25 mg light green and dark green capsules.
	50 mg blue and dark green capsules.

General information
Loxapine is used for the treatment of schizophrenia, mania and other psychotic states. It must be used (if at all) with great caution in patients with heart disease as most patients who take this drug will experience an increased pulse rate. Loxapine must also be used with great caution – if at all – in patients prone to suffering epileptic fits as it can cause fits, even if anticonvulsant drugs are being taken. Loxapine is more dangerous in overdose than other antipsychotic drugs and is described in the British National Formulary as having 'a high potential for serious neurological and cardiac toxicity.' It is said to cause less drowsiness than other antipsychotics.

Dosage information
Adult (16 and over): Treatment begins with 20–50 mg per day taken in two divided doses, which may be increased if necessary over a period of seven to ten days to 60–100 mg daily. In the higher dose range the drug may be taken in three or four divided doses per day. **The maximum dose is 250 mg per day,** which should be reduced to a more normal maintenance dose range of 20–100 mg per day.
Children: Loxapine is not recommended for the treatment of children.

Side effects and further information
Loxapine is similar in its effects to other antipsychotics and may cause weight gain or weight loss, nausea and vomiting, laboured or difficult breathing, blurred vision, trembling limbs, inner restlessness, flushing and headaches. Prolonged use may cause tardive dyskinesia, a condition which causes facial tics and other involuntary movements (for a fuller description of tardive dyskinesia, see pp. 129–130).

METHOTRIMEPRAZINE

Trade name	Description
Nozinan	25 mg white tablets. Ampoules for injection.

General information
Methotrimeprazine is used in the treatment of schizophrenia, mania and other psychotic illnesses. Apart from the fact that it costs about ten times as much chlorpromazine the main difference in effects is that it is more likely to cause sedation, weakness and apathy.

Dosage information
Adult (16 and over): For schizophrenia and psychotic conditions. *By mouth:* Treatment begins with 25–50 mg per day which may be increased or decreased according to the response of the patient. Hospital in-patients may start treatment at between 100–200 mg per day in three divided doses, to be increased or decreased according to the response of the patient. **The maximum dose is 1000 mg per day**. Patients receiving high doses should be kept in bed. When symptoms have been stabilised the dose should be adjusted downward to the minimum dose which controls the symptoms. *By injection:* 12.5–25 mg (in severe agitation up to 50 mg) every 6–8 hours.
Elderly and physically frail: Methotrimeprazine should not be given to people over the age of 50 unless the risk to the patient of a serious reduction in blood pressure has been assessed. Patients with heart problems may be at risk of potentially dangerous effects.
Children: Children are more likely than adults to suffer from the powerful sedating effects of methotrimeprazine. The use of doses

by mouth exceeding 40 mg per day is not recommended by the manufacturers. The usual maintenance dose for a ten-year-old child is said to be between 15 and 20 mg. The use of antipsychotic drugs to treat children is controversial.

Side effects and further information
Methotrimeprazine is also used in the care of terminally ill patients to reduce restlessness and agitation, to increase the effectiveness of pain-relieving drugs and to reduce vomiting. It may cause weight gain or weight loss, nausea and vomiting, laboured or difficult breathing, blurred vision, trembling limbs, inner restlessness, flushing and headaches. Prolonged use may cause tardive dyskinesia, a condition which causes facial tics and other involuntary movements (for a fuller description of tardive dyskinesia and its effects, see pp. 129–130).

OXYPERTINE

Trade name	Description
Under generic name	10 mg white capsules.
	40 mg speckled white tablets.

General information
In low doses oxypertine is used for the short-term treatment of anxiety and depression. In higher doses it is used as a treatment for the symptoms of schizophrenia, mania, other psychotic states and the short-term control of behavioural disturbances. It is claimed to be particularly relevant to the needs of withdrawn schizophrenic patients. In low doses oxypertine is said to cause agitation and hyperactivity and in high doses sedation. In general its effects are broadly similar to chlorpromazine.

Dosage information
Adult (16 and over): *For the short-term treatment of severe anxiety and depression.* Treatment begins with 10 mg three to four times per day after meals, which may be increased or decreased according to the response of the patient. **The maximum dose is 60 mg (six tablets) per day.**

For the treatment of schizophrenia, the short-term management of problem behaviour arising from mental illness and other psychotic states. Treatment begins with 80–120 mg (two or three tablets) per day, which may be increased or decreased according to the response of the patient. **The maximum dose is 300 mg per day**. When control of the symptoms has been achieved the dose should be reduced to the minimum necessary to control the symptoms.

Elderly and physically frail: Doses lower than the normal range of adult doses are recommended.

Children: There are no dose recommendations for children. The use of antipsychotic drugs to treat children is controversial.

Side effects and further information
Oxypertine is broadly similar to chlorpromazine in its actions but is said to cause extrapyramidal side effects less frequently. Prolonged use may cause tardive dyskinesia, a condition which causes facial tics and other involuntary movements (for a fuller description of tardive dyskinesia and its effects, see pp. 129–130).

PERICYAZINE

Trade name	Description
Neulactil	2.5 mg yellow tablets marked Neulactil 2.5.
	10 mg yellow tablets marked Neulactil 10.
	25 mg yellow tablets marked Neulactil 25.
	Brown syrup containing 10 mg per ml.

General information
Pericyazine is used for the treatment of schizophrenia, mania, other psychotic conditions and for the control of problem behaviour in adults and children. Its effects are broadly similar to those of chlorpromazine but it is more likely to cause drowsiness and apathy. At the beginning of treatment reduced blood pressure is common and this may cause patients to feel faint.

Dosage information
Adult: *For the short-term treatment of anxiety, agitation and problem behaviour.* Treatment begins with 15–30 mg per day in two divided doses, the higher dose taken at bedtime, to be increased or decreased according to the patient's response.

For the treatment of schizophrenia, mania and other psychotic states. Treatment begins with 75 mg in divided doses which may be increased if necessary by adding 25 mg to the daily dose at weekly intervals. **The usual maximum dose is 300 mg per day.**

Elderly and physically frail: *For the short-term treatment of severe anxiety.* Treatment begins with 5–10 mg per day divided into two doses with the larger dose taken at bedtime.

For the treatment of schizophrenia, mania and other psychotic states. Treatment begins with 15–30 mg per day which may be increased or decreased according to the response of the patient. Half or quarter the normal adult maintenance dose may be adequate.

Children: *For the control of serious behavioural problems arising from mental illness only.* Treatment begins with 0.5 mg per day for a child with a body weight of 10 kilograms, increased by 1 mg for each additional 5 kilograms of body weight. The dose may be increased or decreased according to the response of the child. The maximum daily dose of 10 mg may be gradually increased but should not exceed twice the starting dose. The use of antipsychotic drugs to treat children is controversial.

Side effects and further information
Pericyazine is more sedating than chlorpromazine and frequently causes a reduction in blood pressure which may cause the patient to feel faint when standing, particularly at the beginning of treatment. Prolonged use may cause tardive dyskinesia, a condition which causes facial tics and other involuntary movements (for a fuller description of tardive dyskinesia and its effects, see pp. 129–130).

PERPHENAZINE

Trade name	Description
Fentazin	2 mg white tablets marked AH/1C.
	4 mg white tablets marked AH/2C.

General information
Perphenazine is used to treat the symptoms of serious mental illnesses such as schizophrenia, mania and other psychotic states of mind. In comparison with chlorpromazine it is said to cause less sedation but much more severe extrapyramidal effects such as muscle spasms in the neck, shoulders and trunk, blurred

vision, dry mouth, stomach upsets and restlessness. Because of the severity of these side effects the drug's manufacturers tell doctors that it should not be used to treat children below the age of 14 or agitated and restless elderly people.

Dosage information
Adult (16 and over): For the treatment of schizophrenia, mania, psychotic states and the control of problem behaviour. Treatment begins with 4 mg three times per day which may be increased or decreased depending on the response of the patient. If necessary the dose can be increased under close supervision to **a maximum dose of 24 mg per day**.
Elderly and physically frail: A quarter to half the normal adult starting dose is suggested by the manufacturers.
Children: Perphenazine should not be given to children below the age of 14. The use of antipsychotic drugs to treat children is controversial.

Side effects and further information
Perphenazine is in the same group of antipsychotic drugs as haloperidol, which is more often prescribed. In very low doses it may be used for the treatment of vomiting and nausea. Prolonged use may cause tardive dyskinesia, a condition which causes facial tics and other involuntary movements (for a fuller description of tardive dyskinesia and its effects, see pp. 129–130).

PIMOZIDE

Trade name	Description
Orap	2 mg white tablets marked JANSSEN.
	4 mg pale green tablets marked JANSSEN.
	10 mg white tablets marked JANSSEN.

General information
Pimozide is one of the newer antipsychotic drugs, having been introduced in Britain in 1971. It is used to treat the same range of symptoms as the other drugs in this class and is suggested to be useful in the treatment of 'monosymptomatic hypochondriacal psychosis'. In other words, for people who believe that they are ill although doctors are unable to find anything wrong with them.

The Government drug watchdog body, the Committee on Safety of Medicines (CSM), has issued a report to doctors drawing their attention to the possible risk of heart damage to patients taking pimozide. Thirteen sudden and unexpected deaths of patients taking the drug have been reported. Seven of these patients were between the ages of 13 and 17. Five of the 13 patients were also taking other antipsychotic drugs (poly-pharmacy) and ten were receiving more than the normal recommended maintenance dose. In their report the Committee suggests that prior to the drug being taken, patients should be given electrocardiographical (ECG) tests to ensure that their hearts are sufficiently robust to receive the drug. Patients receiving in excess of 16 mg per day should regularly have ECG heart checks. The report also warns doctors that the risk of heart damage may be greater if pimozide is used with other antipsychotic drugs. It recommends that substantially lower doses of pimozide should be used than those recommended in the prescribers' handbooks. Since that original CSM report another has been issued suggesting that all patients receiving pimozide should receive an annual electrocardiogram (a test which records the electric activity in the heart as a means to detect problems with its functions).

Dosage information
Adult (16 and over): Treatment with pimozide begins with 10 mg per day. If necessary the dose can be raised in steps of 2–4 mg of one week or more to **the maximum daily dose of 20 mg**. As a treatment to prevent relapse the starting dose is 2 mg per day and maintained at a rate of between 2 and 20 mg per day.
Elderly and physically frail: Pimozide has a long half-life (see below) and elderly people who regularly take it may be prone to levels of the drug building up in their bodies and reaching unintentionally high doses. This exposes elderly people to increased risks of distressing and potentially dangerous side effects, and increases their exposure to the long-term hazards of antipsychotic drugs. The manufacturers recommend that elderly patients should be treated with half the normal starting dose for adults.
Children: Not recommended for the treatment of children.

Side effects and further information
Pimozide has a long 'half-life', which means that it remains in the body of the patient for a longer time than other similar

drugs. This long half-life is not predictable from patient to patient. In some patients the half-life of pimozide is 55 hours whilst for others it is more than 150 hours. When the drug stays in the system for a long period, the patient will begin to accumulate quantities of the drug in the body, which in some patients can lead to overdoses being gradually built up. Prolonged use may cause tardive dyskinesia, a condition which causes involuntary movements of the mouth, face, shoulders, trunk and limbs (for a fuller description of tardive dyskinesia see pp. 129–130).

PROCHLORPERAZINE

Trade name	Description
Buccastem (low-dose preparation for treating vertigo, nausea and vomiting)	3 mg pale yellow tablets.
Under generic name	5 mg white tablets.
Stemetil	5 mg off-white tablets marked Stemetil 5. 25 mg off-white tablets marked Stemetil 25. Injection. 5 mg and 25 mg suppositories. Syrup containing 5 mg per 5 ml.

General information

Prochlorperazine in low-dose preparations is recommended for the treatment of labyrinthitis (an infection of the inner ear); nausea and vomiting from whatever cause including that associated with migraine; schizophrenia (particularly in the chronic stage); acute mania and with other drugs used in the short-term management of anxiety. In high-dose preparations it is recommended for the treatment of schizophrenia and other psychotic disorders.

As an antipsychotic drug, prochlorperazine is said to be less sedating than chlorpromazine but to have more dystonic effects such as muscular spasms in the neck, shoulders and trunk, rigidity and tremors.

Dosage information

Adult (16 and over): *For the treatment of labyrinthitis, vertigo, nausea and vomiting. By mouth:* 5 mg three times per day which may be increased if necessary to **a maximum dose of 30 mg per day**, which may then be gradually reduced to between 5–10 mg per day.

By injection: 12.5 mg injection followed by tablets or syrup after six hours if necessary.

By rectum: 25 mg suppository followed after six hours by tablets or syrup.

For the treatment of the symptoms of schizophrenia, mania and other psychotic conditions.

By mouth: Treatment begins with 12.5 mg twice daily, increased if necessary in steps of 12.5 mg daily and in intervals of between four and twelve days to **the maximum daily dose per day of 75–100 mg**. The dose given may be higher than the maximum in a minority of patients but once the maximum control of symptoms has been achieved the dose should be reduced to the minimum possible to control symptoms.

By injection: Between 12.5 mg and 25 mg twice or three times per day.

By rectum: Suppositories of between 12.5 mg and 25 mg per day, to be changed to tablets or syrup as soon as possible.

Elderly and physically frail: Elderly patients should be started at a lower than normal adult dose. Caution is advised in treating the elderly with this drug as they are more prone to suffer distressing side effects and are more vulnerable to the long-term hazards of antipsychotic drugs.

Children: Prochlorperazine should not be used to treat mental illness in children but in very low doses given in tablet or syrup form it may be used with caution for children with a body weight greater than 10 kilograms, to prevent nausea and vomiting. The manufacturers recommend a dose rate of 0.025 mg per kilogram of body weight per day. With doses of 0.5 mg per kilogram of the child's body weight great caution is recommended because of serious dystonic side effects (see above under General information). Prochlorperazine should not be given to children under 10 kilograms in body weight and should not be administered to any child by injection.

Side effects and further information
Prochlorperazine has been used as an anti-emetic and antipsychotic drug for many years. It has no obvious advantages over the many similar drugs in this group. In the decision of which of the antipsychotics to use, the side effects are usually the deciding factor. Prolonged use may cause tardive dyskinesia, a condition which causes involuntary movements of the mouth, face, shoulders, trunk and limbs (for a fuller description of tardive dyskinesia, see pp. 129–130).

SULPIRIDE

Trade name	Description
Dolmatil	200 mg white tablets marked D200.
Sulparex	200 mg white tablets marked BMS1510.
Sulpitil	200 mg white tablets marked L113.

General information
Sulpiride is chemically different from the other antipsychotic drugs used to treat schizophrenia and other disturbed states of mind and has a number of important differences in its range of effects and side effects. Sulpiride is said by its manufacturers to have antidepressant as well as antipsychotic effects. Where other antipsychotics often make withdrawn patients suffering from schizophrenia even more withdrawn, sulpiride can have the opposite effect of making them more alert. The condition of some seriously agitated 'hypomanic' patients may be aggravated by sulpiride and caution is recommended by the manufacturers with such patients. The risk may be greater if the patient is also taking other medications specifically for the side effects of antipsychotic drugs (for a description of drugs used to treat side effects, see pp. 132–135). Animal research has indicated that the long-term use of sulpiride may be linked to an increased incidence of benign and malignant tumours in the endocrine system. But there is no evidence as yet that such tumours are caused in man.

Dosage information
Adult (16 and over): For patients who are floridly psychotic with hallucinations, thought disorders, delusions, inappropriate emotions and strange fixed ideas. Treatment begins with 400–800 mg per day taken in two divided doses in the morning and early

evening (two or four tablets per day). This may be increased to **the maximum dose of 1200 mg twice daily**. Doses higher than this have not been shown to have any advantages for patients.

For patients who are withdrawn, apathetic, emotionally flat and depressed. Treatment begins with 400 mg twice daily (two tablets in the morning and two in the early evening). If this dose is reduced to 200 mg, the 'alerting' effect is said to be increased. For patients with a mixture of both sets of symptoms listed above the manufacturers recommend a normal dose range of 400–600 mg per day.

Elderly and physically frail: Treatment starts with between 100–400 per day and increased if necessary according to response. Caution in patients with liver disease.

Children: No dosage recommendations are made for children as there is not enough clinical evidence available upon which to base any such recommendations. The use of antipsychotic drugs to treat children is controversial.

Side effects and further information

Sulpiride is one of the most recently introduced antipsychotic drugs, is less sedating than chlorpromazine, and, it is claimed, has fewer and less severe side effects. Sulpiride is less likely to affect the heart than other drugs and does not increase the risk of epileptic fits in people prone to suffering them. Prolonged use may cause tardive dyskinesia, a condition which causes involuntary movements of the mouth, face, shoulders, trunk and limbs (for a fuller description of tardive dyskinesia see pp. 129–130).

THIORIDAZINE

Trade name	Description
Melleril	10 mg white tablets marked 10.
	25 mg white tablets marked 25.
	50 mg white tablets marked 50.
	100 mg white tablets marked 100.
	25 mg per 5 ml spoon creamy-white liquid.
	100 mg per 5 ml spoon creamy-white liquid.
	25 mg per 5 ml spoon orange syrup.
Under generic name	10 mg white tablets.
	25 mg white tablets.
	50 mg white tablets.
	100 mg white tablets.

General information

Thioridazine is used to control the symptoms of schizophrenia, mania, extreme agitation and problem behaviour. It is similar in its effects to chlorpromazine but is less sedating. It should be used with caution in depressed patients as it can aggravate depression. Thioridazine should be avoided in patients who suffer from porphyria, a rare inherited disorder which affects the blood and causes a range of symptoms, such as sensitivity to sunlight, inflammation of the nerves, stomach pain and mental disturbances.

Dosage information

Adult (16 and over): *For schizophrenia, mania and psychotic states.* Treatment begins with 150–600 mg per day in divided doses and may be increased to **the maximum dose of 800 mg per day for hospital in-patients under close specialist supervision**. This high dose should not be given for periods longer than four weeks.

For the control of extreme agitation and dangerous behaviour. Doses between 75–200 mg per day may be given.
Elderly and physically frail: *For the control of agitated restlessness.* Between 30–100 mg per day. Caution is necessary in treating elderly people with antipsychotics, particularly patients who suffer from kidney or liver disease.
Children: Under the age of five, 1 mg per kilogram of body weight daily. Children over the age of five, between 75–300 mg per day to **a maximum dose of 300 mg per day in severe cases**. The use of antipsychotic drugs to treat children is controversial.

Side effects and further information

Thioridazine is a phenothiazine antipsychotic which quite commonly causes reduced blood pressure, making people feel faint. Unlike chlorpromazine, the first drug in this group, thioridazine does not carry a risk of causing jaundice. Prolonged use may cause tardive dyskinesia, a condition which causes involuntary movements of the mouth, face, shoulders, trunk and limbs (for a fuller description of tardive dyskinesia see pp. 129–130).

TRIFLUOPERAZINE

Trade name	Description
Stelazine	1 mg blue tablets marked SKF.
	2 mg clear capsules with yellow caps marked 2.
	5 mg blue tablets marked SKF.
	10 mg clear capsules with yellow caps marked 10.
	15 mg clear capsules with yellow caps marked 15.
	pale yellow peach-flavoured syrup, 1 mg per 5 ml spoon.
	Pale yellow peach-flavoured concentrate containing 10 mg per 1 ml of concentrate.
	Ampoules for injection.
Under generic name	1 mg white tablets.
	5 mg white tablets.

General information

Trifluoperazine is a potent antipsychotic used to control the symptoms of schizophrenia, mania and other psychotic conditions. Its manufacturers claim that it is particularly useful in controlling mania (extreme excitement and agitation). The manufacturers recommend low doses of trifluoperazine for the treatment of depression and anxiety states as it may increase depression rather than relieve it. In common with the other antipsychotics of its type, haloperidol and fluphenazine, trifluoperazine may cause more frequent and more serious extrapyramidal effects: mask-like facial expression, stiffening and trembling of the limbs, pill-rolling movements of the fingers, physical and psychological restlessness, and, occasionally, facial grimaces, an involuntary twisting motion of the neck, and rolling of the eyes. These effects may be treated with other drugs (see pp. 132–135).

Dosage information

Adult (16 and over): *Low dose.* For the short-term treatment of 'anxiety states, depressive symptoms secondary to anxiety, and agitation.' Whatever this says, trifluoperazine may cause these very symptoms. Low-dose treatment begins with 2–4 mg per day given in two doses, morning and early evening. The dose may be increased if necessary to **a maximum dose of 6 mg per day**. At doses higher than this the side effects are likely to be a bigger problem than the one for which the drug was prescribed in the first place.

High dose. For the control of the symptoms of schizophrenia, mania, other psychotic states, the control of severe agitation and problem behaviour. *By mouth:* For physically fit adults treatment begins with 10 mg per day, which can be increased if necessary after one week to 15 mg per day and may be further increased in 5 mg steps at three-day intervals until the symptoms are controlled. When the desired results have been achieved the dose should be gradually reduced to the minimum which provides relief for the patient. **There is no maximum daily dose recommended** by the manufacturers or the publishers of the British National Formulary.

By injection: Treatment begins with 14 mg per day given in two doses. If necessary, the dose may be increased to **a maximum dose of 6 mg per day**. When given by injection the effects and side effects of trifluoperazine are much more rapid and intense. The treatment should be changed from injection to tablets or syrup as soon as possible.

Elderly and physically frail: Treatment should begin with less than half the normal starting dose for fit adults.

Children: *Low dose.* Children aged between three and five, up to 1 mg per day. Children aged between six and twelve, up to **a maximum dose of 4 mg per day**.

High dose. By mouth: Children under 12 should not receive more than **the maximum dose of 5 mg per day in divided doses**. Should a higher dose be considered necessary any increase should be based on an evaluation of the severity of the symptoms being treated and the state of health and body weight of the child. The increase should be done in steps of three-day intervals.

By injection: The manufacturers suggest that doses should be determined on the basis of 1 mg per day per 20 kilograms of the child's body weight. The use of antipsychotic drugs to treat children is controversial.

Side effects and further information

Trifluoperazine is often prescribed in low doses for the treatment of confusion and agitation in the elderly. Even in very low doses some patients experience Parkinsonism, trembling hands, a shuffling walk, an expressionless face and difficulty in movement. Prolonged use may cause tardive dyskinesia, a condition which causes involuntary movements of the mouth, face, shoulders, trunk and limbs (for a fuller description of tardive dyskinesia, see pp. 129–130).

ZUCLOPENTHIXOL ACETATE

Trade name	Description
Clopixol Acuphase	Injection.

General information

Zuclopenthixol acetate is a very powerful and fast-acting antipsychotic drug whose effects last for two to three days. It is used as an emergency treatment to control very agitated people suffering from schizophrenia, mania and other serious psychotic conditions. It should not be used as a maintenance treatment. When a maintenance treatment is required another less powerful drug should be substituted *two days* after the last injection of zuclopenthixol acetate.

Dosage information

Adult: *By deep muscular injection into the backside or the muscular part of the thigh*: 50–150 (**Elderly** 50–100 mg) repeated if necessary after two to three days. One additional dose may be given if necessary one to two days after the first injection. **Maximum cumulative dose 400 mg per course of treatment**. **Maximum number of injections 4**.
Children: Not recommended for children.

Side effects and further information.

Avoid in pregnancy and breast-feeding. Avoid in women of child- bearing age unless they are taking effective contraceptive precautions. Avoid in patients who are sensitive to other antipsychotic drugs. Avoid in patients who are drunk or under the influence of barbiturates, opiates or other narcotics. Avoid in comatose patients. Caution should be exercised in patients who are prone to convulsions, with heart disease, liver or kidney disease. Caution in patients being treated with lithium. Side effects: Sedation, drowsiness, dry mouth, stuffy nose, lightheadedness due to reduced blood pressure when standing. Blurred vision, impotence, difficulty in urinating, constipation and Parkinsonism. For a full description of side effects, see p. 125).

ZUCLOPENTHIXOL DIHYDROCHLORIDE

Trade name	Description
Clopixol	2 mg pink tablets.
	10 mg light brown tablets.
	25 mg brown tablets.

General information

Zuclopenthixol is a potent, rapidly acting antipsychotic drug used to control the symptoms of schizophrenia, mania and other psychotic states and for the emergency control of dangerous behaviour. Particularly in the early stages of treatment the side effects may be severe. The side effects include lethargy, depression, loss of motivation, muscular rigidity and tremors. Where necessary these side effects may be reduced by other medications (for details of medication for side effects, see pp. 132–135).

Dosage information

Adult: Treatment begins with 20–30 mg per day which may be increased to a maximum dose of 150 mg per day in divided doses. The usual maintenance dose is between 20–50 mg per day which should be reduced if possible.
Elderly: Lower doses should be considered in elderly or frail people.
Children: Not recommended for the treatment of children.

Side effects and further information

Zuclopenthixol should not be used in the treatment of withdrawn or apathetic patients. Prolonged use may cause tardive dyskinesia, a condition which causes involuntary movements of the mouth, face, shoulders, trunk and limbs (for a fuller description of tardive dyskinesia, see pp. 129–130).

Antipsychotic depot injections

The compounds described in this section are used to treat patients who may be reluctant or who forget to take their antipsychotic drugs. The drugs may be injected on a weekly, fortnightly, three-weekly or monthly basis. Most patients who are maintained on depot antipsychotics receive their injections monthly. It is often difficult to establish the dose which gives the individual the maximum relief of symptoms with the minimum of side effects. This means that it is often necessary to supplement the depot injection of the antipsychotic with other non-depot preparations until the appropriate dose for an individual patient has been established. As depot antipsychotics are often very powerful care and sensitivity should be exercised in their use. Sadly such care is not always evident. Some depot injection clinics operate as production lines which require the minimum effort from the nurses and psychiatrists who run them. This is community care delivered by syringe – the battery farming of people rather than services designed to respond to their individual and changing needs.

Depot antipsychotic injections should not be routinely given at the same time as antipsychotic pills and syrups, but they often are. Care should be taken to establish the lowest possible dose necessary to control symptoms, but often it is not. Antipsychotic drugs should not be routinely prescribed in cocktails with antidepressant drugs, but they often are. The side effects of depot antipsychotic injections are often more frequent and more severe than those of antipsychotic pills. Many patients are given high doses of depot antipsychotics over long periods of time with the most minimal review of their needs. Such practices expose patients to more severe life-diminishing side effects and increased risks of developing tardive dyskinesia and dopamine supersensitivity. Fifty per cent of patients maintained on depot antipsychotics suffer from tardive dyskinesia compared to 20–40 per cent maintained on oral medications. Just how many long term patients who are now more likely to suffer from serious psychotic symptoms as a direct consequence of dopamine supersensivity caused by their medication is probably not known.

People being treated with depot antipsychotics should insist that their medication needs are regularly reviewed. Relatives and carers should support patients in pressing for such reviews.

Some patients will be unable to press for such reviews, either because they are so sedated that they are effectively disabled, or because nobody will listen to them.

Depot antipsychotics have an almost unique potential for abuse. Whilst they can relieve the torment of the symptoms of serious mental illness for many people, they can also reduce an individual to an unprotesting zombie-like state. For some patients the use of depot antipsychotics is little more than an exchange of one form of human misery for another. Drowsiness, lethargy, loss of motivation, impotence, stiffened muscles, shaking hands, physical restlessness, severe anxiety and persistent constipation may be more distressing to some people than a fixed belief that their thoughts are being controlled by the international brotherhood of Freemasons. For others these side effects are a small price to pay for the relief that the drugs give them from a much more distressing and terrifying psychotic inner reality.

Starting on a course of antipsychotic depot injections is a major watershed in the life of an individual. For many it may be the start of a lifetime career as a mental patient attending a depot clinic for injections and a day centre to pack pencils into boxes for cigarette money. Getting the antipsychotic dose right for a particular patient can be difficult. It is very much easier to prescribe these powerful drugs in high doses which make the patient less demanding and more manageable. The quality of the services provided in Britain's mental hospitals and depot clinics varies enormously. Johnson and Wright (1990)[8] in their study of prescribing practices in the treatment of schizophrenia stressed the need for 'constant vigilance in supervising the depot injection clinics'. MIND heartily supports this view.

Five-point guide to getting the most from antipsychotic depot injections

1. Antipsychotic depot drugs should not be routinely prescribed but used only when oral drugs have been shown to be inappropriate to the needs of the individual patient.

[8] Johnson, D.A.W. and Wright, N.F., 'Drug Prescribing for Schizophrenic Out Patients on Depot Injections. Repeat Surveys over 18 years,' *British Journal of Psychiatry*, 56 (1990), 827–34.

2. Antipsychotic depot drugs should be prescribed in the lowest possible dose that meets the medical and social needs of the patient.

3. When depot antipsychotics are prescribed all other antipsychotics should be stopped.

4. The doses of depot antipsychotic drugs should be regularly reviewed with the patient and adjusted to the minimum required in the circumstances.

5. Depot antipsychotics should not be used to treat children or confused elderly people, patients under the influence of alcohol or other drugs which have a depressant action on the central nervous system, patients who suffer from Parkinsonism, or any patient with a known sensitivity to antipsychotic drugs.

FLUPENTHIXOL DECANOATE
(trade name Depixol)

General information
Flupenthixol decanoate is used in the maintenance control of the symptoms of schizophrenia and other psychotic conditions. It is given by deep intramuscular injection into the buttock, which may be painful and cause swelling and small lumps at the site of the injection. The injection may be given once a fortnight or once a month.

Dosage information
Adult (16 and over): A trial dose of 20 mg should be given to assess the patient's response to the drug before the treatment is started. If the drug causes the patient no serious adverse reactions, the treatment should begin five to ten days after the test dose with a further dose of between 20–40 mg, repeated at intervals of two to four weeks. The dose may be lowered or increased depending on the response of the patient. **The maximum dose is 400 mg per four weeks**. The usual maintenance dosage range is from 50 mg every four weeks to 300 mg every two weeks. The progress of the patient should be very closely reviewed, with a view to reducing the dose as soon as is practically possible.
Elderly and physically frail: Elderly people should start treatment with a quarter of the normal starting dose. Elderly and physically frail people are more prone to suffering from distressing side effects.
Children: Not recommended for the treatment of children.

Side effects and further information

Flupenthixol may have a mood-lifting or alerting effect and so may be more helpful to depressed and withdrawn patients; it may cause violent or aggressive behaviour in agitated patients. If such a response occurs it may be necessary to change to another antipsychotic compound. The side effects of the drug occur within one to five days of the injection and reduce in severity after about five days. The side effects include lethargy, loss of motivation, muscular rigidity, tremors, physical restlessness, blurred vision, dry mouth and a mask-like facial expression. Where necessary these side effects may be reduced by other medications (for details of medications for side effects, see pp. 132–135). Prolonged use may cause tardive dyskinesia, a condition which causes involuntary movements of the mouth, face, shoulders, trunk and limbs (for a fuller description of tardive dyskinesia, see pp. 129–130).

FLUPHENAZINE DECANOATE

(trade name Modecate)

General information

Fluphenazine decanoate is used in the maintenance control of the symptoms of schizophrenia and other psychotic conditions. It is administered by deep intramuscular injection into the buttock. The injection may be given at regular intervals of between 14 and 35 days.

Dosage information

Adult (16 and over): Before the treatment is started a trial dose of 12.5 mg should be given to assess the patient's response to the drug. If the drug is well tolerated, after an interval of between four and seven days a dose of between 12.5–100 mg may be given and repeated at intervals of 14 to 35 days. The dose may be adjusted upwards or downwards according to the response of the patient. **Maximum dose 100 mg per 14 days**. As can be seen, the dose range of this drug is very wide, with the highest recommended dose eight times that of the lowest. The progress of patients should be very closely reviewed, with a view to reducing the dose as soon as is practically possible.

Elderly and physically frail: Elderly people should receive a trial dose of 6.25 mg (half the usual trial dose) and be treated with lower doses. Elderly and physically frail people are more prone to suffering from distressing side effects.

Children: Not recommended for the treatment of children.

Side effects and further information

Fluphenazine should not be prescribed to patients who are severely depressed as it may seriously worsen the depression. It may take some days for the antipsychotic action of fluphenazine to take effect. Within hours of the injection extrapyramidal side effects may be experienced, such as a mask-like facial appearance, stiffening of limbs, inability to sit or stand still, blurred vision and loss of motivation. Prolonged use may cause tardive dyskinesia, a condition which causes involuntary movements of the mouth, face, shoulders, trunk and limbs (for a fuller description of tardive dyskinesia see pp. 129–130). Where necessary these side effects may be reduced by other medications (for details of medications for side effects, see pp. 132–135).

FLUSPIRILINE
(trade name Redeptin)

General information

Fluspiriline is used for the control of the symptoms of schizophrenia and other psychotic conditions. It is administered by deep intramuscular injection into the buttock, which may be painful and cause swelling and small lumps at the site of the injection. Fluspiriline is said to be less sedating than chlorpromazine and its side effects are said to compare favourably with other antipsychotic drugs used in similar doses.

Dosage information

Adult (16 and over): Treatment begins with 2 mg per week, which may be increased in weekly increases of 2 mg until the desired response has been achieved. The usual maintenance dose is between 2–8 mg and **the maximum dose is 20 mg per week**. The progress of patients should be very closely reviewed, with a view to reducing the dose as soon as is practically possible.

Elderly and physically frail: Elderly people should begin treatment with a quarter to half the normal dose. Elderly and physically frail people are more prone to suffering from distressing side effects.

Children: Not recommended for the treatment of children.

Side effects and further information

It may take some weeks before psychotic symptoms are relieved by fluspiriline. Common side effects are restlessness and sweating. Prolonged use may cause tardive dyskinesia, a condition which causes involuntary movements of the mouth, face, shoulders, trunk and limbs (for a fuller description of tardive dyskinesia, see pp. 129–130). Where necessary these side effects may be reduced by other medications (for details of medications for side effects, see pp. 132–135).

HALOPERIDOL DECANOATE

(trade name Haldol decanoate)

General information

Haloperidol decanoate is used for the maintenance control of schizophrenia and other psychotic conditions. It is administered by deep intramuscular injection into the buttock, which may be painful and cause swelling and small lumps at the site of the injection. It is less sedating than chlorpromazine but its other side effects may be more severe and more frequent.

Dosage information

Adult (16 and over): Treatment begins with 50 mg every four weeks which if necessary may be increased after two weeks in steps of 50 mg to the usual **maximum dose of 300 mg per four weeks**. A small number of patients may be given higher doses. The progress of patients should be very closely reviewed, with a view to reducing the dose as soon as is practically possible.

Elderly and physically frail: Treatment begins with low doses (12.5 mg). Elderly and physically frail people are more prone to suffering from distressing side effects.

Children: Not recommended for the treatment of children.

Side effects and further information

Haloperidol is less sedating than chlorpromazine but is more likely to cause extrapyramidal side effects such as inner agitation, physical restlessness, a mask-like facial appearance, tremors and muscular rigidity. Prolonged use may cause tardive dyskinesia, a condition which causes facial tics and other involuntary movements of the shoulders, trunk and limbs (for a fuller description of tardive dyskinesia, see pp. 129–130). Where necessary these side effects may be reduced by other medications (for details of medications for side effects, see pp. 132–135).

PIPOTHIAZINE PALMITATE

(trade name Piportil Depot)

General information

Pipothiazine is used for the maintenance control of schizophrenia and other psychotic conditions. It is administered by deep intramuscular injection into the buttocks, which may be painful and cause swelling and small lumps at the site of the injection. Pipothiazine is said to have a moderately sedative action compared with chlorpromazine, to which it is related. This drug should be avoided in depressed patients as it may make the depression more severe.

Dosage information

Adult (16 and over): Before treatment begins a trial dose of 25 mg should be given to test the patient's reaction to the drug. If the drug is well tolerated, after an interval of between four and seven days a dose of between 25–50 mg may be given and repeated at intervals of four weeks. The dose may be increased or decreased according to the response of the patient. **Maximum dose 200 mg per 4 weeks**. The progress of patients should be very closely reviewed, with a view to reducing the dose as soon as is practically possible.

Elderly and physically frail: Treatment begins with 12.5 mg (half the usual starting dose). Elderly and physically frail people are more prone to suffering from distressing side effects.

Children: Not recommended for the treatment of children.

Side effects and further information

Pipothiazine may cause severe Parkinsonism, a slowing of movements, stiffened arms, tremors, an expressionless facial appearance and some people's fingers may make a 'pill-rolling' movement. Prolonged use may cause tardive dyskinesia, a condition which causes involuntary movements of the mouth, face, shoulders, trunk and limbs (for a fuller description of tardive dyskinesia, see pp. 129–130). Where necessary these side effects may be reduced by other medications (for details of medications for side effects, see pp. 132–135).

ZUCLOPENTHIXOL DECANOATE.
(trade name Clopixol)

General information
Zuclopenthixol decanoate is used for the maintenance control of schizophrenia and other psychotic conditions. It is administered by deep intramuscular injection into the buttocks, which may be painful and cause swelling and small lumps at the site of the injection. Zuclopenthixol should be avoided in porphyria, a rare inherited disorder caused by a disturbance in the way the body deals with the breakdown products of red blood cells. The disorder may be in the bone marrow, the liver or in both. The symptoms of porphyria are: sensitivity to sunlight, causing inflammation and blisters, blue urine, inflammation of the nerves, mental disturbances, and attacks of abdominal pain. A form of porphyria is also associated with chronic alcoholism.

Dosage information
Adult (16 and over): Before treatment begins a trial dose of 100 mg should be given to test the patient's reaction to the drug. If the drug is well tolerated, after an interval of between 7 and 28 days a dose of 100–200 mg or more may be given, followed at intervals of two to four weeks by doses of 200–400 mg. **The maximum dose is 600 mg per week**. The dose may be increased or decreased according to the response of the patient. The progress of patients should be very closely reviewed, with a view to reducing the dose as soon as is practically possible.
Elderly and physically frail: It is recommended that elderly people should be treated with one-fifth of the normal dose. Elderly and physically frail people are more prone to suffering from distressing side effects.
Children: Not recommended for the treatment of children.

Side effects and further information
Zuoclopenthixol is said to be useful for the treatment of agitated or aggressive patients. It is said to be less sedating than chlorpromazine, to have fewer extrapyramidal side effects, but to cause more Parkinsonism-like side effects. Prolonged use may cause tardive dyskinesia, a condition which causes involuntary movements of the mouth, face, shoulders, trunk and limbs (for a fuller description of tardive dyskinesia, see pp. 129–130).

Antipsychotic drugs: side effects and further information

The following list of side effects applies to all the antipsychotic drugs listed in this guide. There are, however, differences between some of the drugs in the severity and frequency with which the side effects occur. Another complicating factor is that antipsychotic drugs affect different people in different ways and some people are much more likely than others to find side effects distressing. Elderly and physically frail people are much more vulnerable to serious side effects than those who are younger and fitter. Two other factors also affect the severity of the side effects:

The dose: The higher the dose, the more frequent and more severe will be the side effects. In higher doses antipsychotics are more likely to cause tardive dyskinesia (see pp. 129–130).

The number of drugs taken: The more different drugs taken, the more frequent and more severe will be the side effects. The combination of antidepressants with antipsychotics enhances the side effects of both drugs. Such combinations also increase the risk of tardive dyskinesia as tricyclic antidepressants are very closely related to phenothiazine antipsychotics and have many similar effects. The medications given to relieve the side effects of antipsychotic drugs also increase the risk of tardive dyskinesia.

The best results for the patient are achieved when antipsychotic drugs are used at the lowest effective dose for the needs of the individual patient and when they are used with as few other drugs as possible.

If you are troubled by side effects you should notify the prescribing doctor and, if necessary, not hesitate to make a nuisance of yourself until you are satisfied that the drugs and doses prescribed have been tailored to your own particular needs.

Side effects – how serious and how common?

Antipsychotic drugs do not have exactly the same effects and side effects for everyone and many of them vary depending on the dose given. Some patients require higher doses to obtain relief of symptoms than others. Some people suffer from the side effects of antipsychotic drugs more severely and at lower doses than others. Elderly people, the physically frail and children are more likely to be troubled side effects. People taking antipsychotic drugs frequently become lethargic and lose motivation which means that they may not complain about side effects unless they are specifically asked about them. When patients are generally asked questions about their treatment, the side effects of drugs feature very prominently amongst their concerns. The experience of side effects is first and foremost a subjective experience which is extremely difficult, if not impossible, to measure scientifically. It is generally accepted that the adverse effects of prescribed drugs are under-reported. The prescribers' handbooks do give some broad indications as to the frequency of the side effects of individual drugs, but the reliability of such indications is suspect. They assume a level of sensitivity on the part of the prescribers which is simply not evident in psychiatry. An abundance of anecdotal evidence and a substantial amount of published evidence points to prescribing practices which fall far short of anything which might be described as sensitive.

The purpose of this guide is not to reassure people about the effects of psychiatric drugs or to encourage them to take them, but to validate their experiences and empower them in informed discussions with their doctors. For these reasons the side effects listed below are not classified according to their frequency or their severity. However, it should be remembered that not everyone will experience or be troubled by all of the side effects listed below. When consent is being sought for a drug treatment the issue of side effects should be dealt with candidly and frankly, otherwise that consent is of dubious legality. The worries of the person whose consent is being sought should be listened to and dealt with properly. Quite often in the hurly-burly of the hospital or clinic the consent of the patient is assumed rather than asked for. People subject to detention under the Mental Health Act may in certain circumstances be treated without their consent (see pp. 151–155). The rest of us have a legal right not to be treated without our consent. We have a responsibility to ourselves and to one another to protect that right by exercising it. By so doing we can play a real part in protecting our health and in improving the quality of the services we receive when we need them.

Side effects of antipsychotics
Unless otherwise stated, all the side effects listed below are only a problem whilst the drugs are being taken.

Eyes: Blurred vision. Miosis (narrowing of the pupil). Perphenazine and trifluoperazine can cause mydriasis (widening of the pupil). With long-term use, the pigmentation may occur in the retina, conjunctiva and cornea of the eye, which can impair vision.

Stomach and bladder: Constipation. Decreased secretion of gastric fluids and reduced reflex movements of the stomach. Decreased saliva (dry mouth). Nausea. Rarely, reduced urination.

Sexual functions: Reduced sexual arousal. Difficulty in achieving orgasm. Impotence. Sterility. Menstrual periods may become irregular or stop. Galactorrhoea (the production of milk in the breasts). Rarely, gynaecomastia (abnormal enlargement of the breasts in men), priaprism (a persistent involuntary erection of the penis which may require surgical treatment), a reduction in the size and weight of testicles.

Body temperature regulation: Patients on antipsychotics are more vulnerable to hypothermia (reduced body temperature) in cold weather and hyperthermia (increased body temperature) in hot weather.

Brain: 'Pseudo-Parkinsonism', which can cause a mask-like facial expression, muscular rigidity, shaking hands, disturbed balance, stiffening of the neck, a shuffling walk (often referred to in Britain as the 'Modecate' or 'Largactil shuffle' and in the US as the 'Prolixin stomp'), apathy and depression. Approximately one-third of patients treated with normal doses of antipsychotic drugs will be affected by pseudo-Parkinsonism. Reduced seizure threshold, increasing the risk of epileptic fits in people prone to suffering them. When high doses are used, there is a risk that people with no previous history of or disposition to epileptic seizures may suffer fits. Nightmares. Insomnia. Akathisia (inner agitation and restlessness, anxiety and an inability to sit or stand still). Tardive dyskinesia (see pp. 129–130), a condition which appears to be permanent in many patients. Long-term use may cause dopamine receptor (nerve cells in the brain involved in the transmission of messages) supersensitivity, which may cause a worsening of the symptoms of schizophrenia when antipsychotic drugs are withdrawn.

Skin: Photosensitivity (increased risk of sunburn after moderate exposure). Pallor. Sweating. With long-term use, purplish pigmentation of the skin. Rashes. One in twenty patients may expect to suffer skin problems. With injected antipsychotics, small nodules may appear at the site of the injections. Jaundice (see below), which causes a characteristic yellow skin tint.

Liver: Obstructive jaundice (a form of jaundice caused by the obstruction of bile ducts).

Autoimmune system: Very rarely, a condition resembling lupus erythematosus, a disease which affects the skin and internal organs. The most common sign is a red scaly rash on the face, affecting the nose and cheeks, arthritis and progressive damage to the kidney. In its mildest forms only the skin is affected. It can render patients more prone to catching infections.

Heart, circulation and blood: Reduced blood pressure which can cause the patient to feel faint when standing. Occasionally patients may faint. Changes in rate of heart beat. Pimozide has been associated with sudden deaths, which are caused by its effects on the heart (see p. 107). Agranulocytosis (a condition in which damage to the bone marrow causes a serious deficiency of white blood cells). Although this condition is very rare (it is estimated that one in 10,000 patients will suffer it), it may lead rapidly to collapse and death. Another rare side effect is haemolytic anaemia (the destruction of red blood cells).

Body weight: Weight gain, which can be substantial.

The neuroleptic malignant syndrome: The neuroleptic malignant syndrome (NMS) is a rare and potentially fatal side effect of antipsychotic drugs whose exact cause is unknown. Of patients who are affected by NMS approximately one in five die. Studies into the frequency of NMS put the risk between two and ten patients per thousand, but these figures may be an overestimate. The symptoms of NMS include changing states of consciousness, rapidly increased body temperature, muscular rigidity, pale skin, increased heart rate, urinary incontinence, changes in breathing and sweating. There is no treatment which has been proved to be effective for NMS. The condition appears to last for as long as the antipsychotic drug remains in the body; for between five and ten days with tablets, syrup, or short-term injections, but two weeks or longer with depot preparations.

Tardive dyskinesia

Translated from the Latin, tardive dyskinesia means involuntary movement of late onset and constitutes the most common and most worrying hazard associated with the use of antipsychotic drugs. The symptoms of TD are:

Facial movements. A constant sucking of the lips. Movements of the jaw from side to side with the mouth partially open. Darting, 'fly-catching' and rolling movements of the tongue. Frowning or raising of the eyebrows. Grimacing. Increased blinking and rolling of the eyes.

Movements of the neck and shoulders. A rolling motion of the neck and a persistent, slow rolling and shrugging movement of the shoulders.

Movements of the limbs. Spreading, twisting and 'piano playing' movements of the fingers. Spreading movements of the toes. Foot tapping and a rotating movement of the ankles.

Movements of the trunk. Pelvic thrusting movement.

Breathing and swallowing movements. Disturbances in breathing rhythm which may be accompanied by animal-like grunting noises. Swallowing may be difficult.

These movements are beyond the person's control and tend to disappear whilst he or she is asleep. They are usually first noticed when antipsychotic drugs are reduced in dose or withdrawn. The only effective way to control them is by administering more of the drug which caused them in the first place and thus exposing the patient to the risk of making the underlying condition worse. In its most severe and extremely rare form, TD can be a crippling condition.

A small minority of psychiatrists doubt that TD is caused by antipsychotic drugs. They point to the fact that Emil Kraepelin, the psychiatrist who first classified the group of symptoms which we now call schizophrenia, described involuntary movements similar to those of TD in his patients at the beginning of the century, long before the discovery of chlorpromazine, the first antipsychotic drug. However, the main body of opinion is that TD is caused by antipsychotic drugs, usually after years of use of the drugs but very rarely after a single dose.

It is very difficult to predict the statistical risk of contracting TD: estimates of its prevalence vary from just over 5 per cent of people receiving long-term treatment with antipsychotic drugs to as high as 56 per cent. This wide discrepancy arises because different researchers have used different criteria to define TD. The most widely accepted figure for the number of people who are treated with antipsychotics for periods of three years or longer and who develop TD is 20 per cent, or one in five. The risk of TD is thought to be highest for elderly patients and in particular for elderly female patients. Women patients tend to be treated with higher doses of antipsychotic drugs than men, so this increased risk of TD may well be a reflection of this factor, rather than of any gender-related biological differences between men and women. Although the elderly do seem to be at more risk of suffering TD, it is reported in younger patients, including adolescents. Another major risk factor in TD is the dose of antipsychotics taken, the higher the dose the greater the risk of being affected. Patients on depot injections appear to be more at risk than those on oral preparations. The anti-Parkinsonism drugs used to treat the side effects of antipsychotic drugs may also increase the risk of TD.

TD has been described in medical literature as a 'major public health hazard' and 'probably the most commonly diagnosed iatrogenic (a condition caused by treatment) disorder of the central nervous system'. A training video called 'Tardive Dyskinesia Observed', produced for doctors by the Newcastle Medical School, estimates that 40 per cent of all chronic (long-term) patients treated with antipsychotics have TD to some degree. TD has come to be regarded as the stigmata of the modern psychiatric patient.

Tardive dyskinesia can seriously diminish a person's quality of life, and his or her prospects of resuming a valued role in the community. The short-term side effects of antipsychotic drugs alone are sufficiently serious to merit the greatest degree of care in the way they are prescribed and used. TD adds urgency to the need for sensitivity in the prescribing practices in psychiatry. A number of people diagnosed as schizophrenic will not suffer symptoms of sufficient severity to justify the use of antipsychotic drugs. Others will not relapse for many years after their first episode and others will have experienced only an episode. In an ideal world such patients and their relatives should be offered a trial of drug-free management of symptoms. Some interesting and encouraging work has been done using cognitive psychology to manage symptoms. There is also good evidence that various forms of milieu therapy can be effective. But the pre-eminence of pharmaceuticals in psychiatry has effectively ruled these out for most of us.

HOW ANTIPSYCHOTICS INTERACT WITH OTHER DRUGS AND MEDICINES

Alcohol	Increased sedation.
Anaesthetics	Increased reduction of blood pressure.
Indomethacin painkillers such as Flexin Continus; Indocid & Indocid-R, Indocid PDA, Indolar SR, Indomod, Rheumacinla, Slo-Indo. Antacids	Severe drowsiness when given with haloperidol. Reduced absorption of phenothiazines.
Rifampicin antibacterial drugs such as Rifadin, Rifater ,Rifinah 150 and 300, Rimactane, Rimactazid 150 and 300	Haloperidol is metabolised more quickly, which reduces the amount of haloperidol in the blood, thereby reducing its effects.
Tricyclic antidepressants	Increased side effects of phenothiazines.
MAOI antidepressants	Increased blood pressure and excitation with oxypertine (Integrin).
Anti-epileptics	Antipsychotics reduce the effectiveness of anti-epileptic drugs. Carbamazepine (Tegretol, Tegretol Retard) increases the rate at which haloperidol is metabolised.
Drugs used to reduce blood pressure	Increased reduction of blood pressure. Increased risk of extrapyramidal side effects with methyldopa (Aldomet, Dopamet), metirosine (Demser).
Antimuscarinic drugs, for example drugs used to treat bronchitis, such as Atrovent, Rinatec. Drugs used to treat side effects of antipsychotics such as Artane, Cogentin, Disipal, Kemadrin. Also drugs used in the treatment of bladder and stomach disorders	Reduces the concentration of phenothiazine antipsychotics. May increase the likelihood of tardive dyskinesia. Increased extrapyramidal side effects. If the patient has tardive dyskinesia this will be 'unmasked'.
Tranquillisers and sleeping pills	Increased drowsiness and sedation.

Conditions in which antipsychotic drugs should be avoided
Comatose patients. People who are drunk or under the influence
of narcotics. Bone marrow deficiencies. Glaucoma (a condition
in which pressure in the eye is abnormally high). See also the list-
ings for individual drugs.

*Conditions in which antipsychotic drugs should be used with
caution*
Old age (70 and over). Heart disease. Diseases of the blood vessels in the brain. Respiratory diseases (pneumonia, pleurisy,
severe bronchitis). Phaeochromocytoma (a tumour in the
adrenal gland which causes increased blood pressure and heart
rate, palpitations and headaches). Parkinsonism. Epilepsy. Serious infections. Pregnancy. Breast-feeding. Liver disease. Kidney
disease. History of jaundice. Leucopenia (a reduction in the
white blood cells). Hypothyroidism (a reduced function of the
thyroid gland, causing reduced metabolism, tiredness and
lethargy). Myasthenia gravis (a chronic disease marked by severe
fatigue and muscular weakness which can cause temporary
paralysis). Enlarged prostate gland (common in older men).
Caution should be exercised in elderly or frail people in very hot
or cold weather. Patients given intramuscular injections should
remain lying down for 30 minutes after receiving the injection.

Drugs for the treatment of the
side effects of antipsychotics
(anti-Parkinsonism drugs)

As this guide shows, all antipsychotic drugs have a wide range of
serious, unwanted effects which are often sufficiently distressing
to warrant treatment in their own right, and amongst these
'pseudo-Parkinsonism' may be the most troublesome. The drugs
used to treat these side effects are the same as the drugs used to
treat Parkinsonism and are referred to as anticholinergics or
antimuscarinics, but for the sake of simplicity and clarity the
term used in this guide is anti-Parkinsonism drugs. These drugs
have their own unwanted effects and problems associated with
their use, and although they can reduce some of the side effects
of antipsychotics, they do so at a price. That price is the
exchange of one set of unwanted effects for another, hopefully
more tolerable, set of side effects and an increased exposure to

the risk of tardive dyskinesia. High doses of antipsychotics increase the severity and frequency of their side effects. Patients on high doses are therefore more likely to be given medication for the control of side effects, and as a consequence they are also at greater risk of suffering permanent damage to their central nervous system. Antipsychotic drugs can actually mask tardive dyskinesia, but it is usually revealed when the dose of antipsychotic is reduced or the drug stopped. It may also be revealed by anti-Parkinsonism medication.

Anti-Parkinsonism drugs are often routinely administered with antipsychotic drugs, which is extremely controversial. The World Health Organisation recently issued a consensus statement on the use of anti-Parkinsonism drugs in which the arguments against their routine use was summarised as follows:

'(a) The long-term use of anticholinergics may predispose to tardive dyskinesia (in fact, the administration of these agents exacerbates the syndrome in affected patients and has been used as an aid to its early detection). (b) Anticholinergic medication may induce autonomic side effects, which may be sometimes serious (urinary retention, paralytic ileus). (c) The long-term use of anticholinergics is likely to affect memory functions, and thus further compromise the already impaired cognitive performance of schizophrenic patients. (d) It has been suggested that anticholinergics may contribute to the development of hyperthermic episodes, some of which may be fatal. (e) The consumption of an excessive dose of anticholinergics may produce an acute toxic state, with agitation, disorientation in time and space, delusions and hallucinations. (f) In some cases, anticholinergics may be abused as euphoriants, so that their discontinuation may be difficult. (g) There are some indications that anticholinergics can decrease the therapeutic activity of neuroleptics, although early reports of pharmacokinetic interactions between the two classes of drugs have not been confirmed by more recent studies. (h) Many patients on antipsychotic therapy do not develop Parkinsonism, so that preventative treatment is sometimes useless.'

The WHO consensus statement concludes: 'On the basis of these considerations, the prophylactic use of anticholinergics in patients on neuroleptic treatment is not recommended, and may be justified only early in treatment (after which it should be discontinued and its need should be re-evaluated). As a rule these compounds should only be used when Parkinsonism has actually developed, and when other measures, such as the reduction of neuroleptic dosage or the substitution of the administered drug by another less prone to induce Parkinsonism, have proven ineffective.'

DRUGS USED TO TREAT THE SIDE EFFECTS OF ANTIPSYCHOTIC DRUGS

Generic name	Trade name	Description	Dose
Benzhexol	**Artane**	2 mg white tablets marked Lederle 4434. 5 mg white tablets marked Lederle 4436.	Treatment begins with 1 mg (half a tablet) per day, taken before or after meals, and gradually increased to the usual maintenance dose of between 5–15 mg per day in three to four divided doses.
	Broflex	Pink syrup containing 5 mg per 5 ml.	
	Benzhexol (generic)	2 mg white tablets. 5 mg white tablets.	
Orphenadrine hydrochloride	**Biorphen**	Elixir containing 25 mg per 5ml.	150 mg per day in divided doses before or after meals which may be gradually increased to a maximum dose of 400 mg per day.
	Disipal	50 mg yellow tablets.	
Procyclidine hydrochloride	**Arpicolin**	Syrup containing 2.5 mg per ml.	Usual daily dose for the control of antipsychotic drug side effects 20: mg.
	Kemadrin	5 mg white tablets marked WELLCOME S3A. Injection.	
	Procyclidine (generic)	5 mg white tablets.	

General information

These drugs are used for the treatment of Parkinsonism and the side effects of antipsychotic drugs. In higher doses they have a stimulating effect. These drugs should not be routinely prescribed with antipsychotics. Normally they should be stopped after three to four months and the patient's continuing need for them should be reviewed.

Side effects and further information

These drugs should be avoided in patients suffering urinary retention, glaucoma and blocked intestines. Avoid in patients with tardive dyskinesia. It should be used with caution in patients with heart, kidney or liver disease. Should not be withdrawn abruptly. These drugs have a potential to be used recreationally; patients have been known to hoard this drug in order to get 'high' on them. An overdose can produce euphoria, aural and visual hallucinations.

PART FOUR

Antimanic Drugs

Introduction

Manic depression is characterised by moods which swing dramatically between the depths of depression and euphoric 'highs'. It can appear without warning, and occasionally it vanishes just as mysteriously. In the depressed phase of the illness the sufferer sinks to the lowest despair and in the manic phase is driven by euphoric flights of fantasy. Between periods of deep depression and mania the individual will lead a perfectly ordinary and unremarkable life. Many sufferers are creative and successful people, but many more live on a razor's edge of potential disaster. In the depressive phase the sufferer may be suicidally depressed. In the manic phase he or she may be abnormally and destructively sexually promiscuous, or driven to making disastrous financial decisions by unshakeable beliefs in fantasy opportunities. Antipsychotic drugs are often used to bring people down from their psychotic highs, with antidepressants used to treat their depression. Lithium is used to stabilise and prevent these mood swings and for about 70 per cent of people who suffer from manic depression it is very successful.

The lightest of all metals, lithium is a naturally occurring element which was discovered in 1817. It has been used to treat a wide variety of conditions. In the middle of the last century it was used as a treatment for gout, in the 1920s as a sleeping draught and in the 1940s as a sodium substitute. This therapeutic pragmatism with lithium had disastrous and frequently fatal consequences. Lithium was first tried as a treatment for manic depression in 1949 by an Australian called Cade. In the course of some experiments, Cade noticed that guinea pigs became lethargic when injected with lithium. From this observation he took a mighty leap in the dark and gave it to ten manic depressive patients. In 1949 he published his paper showing that all ten patients had benefited from lithium. However, at that time there was little interest in the psychiatric community in Cade's findings. Lithium's disastrous track record was against it. Psychiatry at that time was about to embark on its honeymoon with chlorpromazine, the first of the antipsychotics. Cade's discovery did not fire the imagination of psychiatry or the pharmaceutical industry. It was not until 1968, when a Danish psychiatrist called Schou reported positive findings in the prevention of both depressive and manic phases of the illness, that lithium began to gain respectability as a useful treatment.

Just how lithium exerts its effects on manic depression remains a matter of theory and speculation. How and why it stabilises mood remains as mysterious as the workings of most other psychiatric drugs and electro-convulsive therapy. Lithium is one of the most toxic substances used in medicine and the dividing line between its therapeutic and toxic doses is very narrow indeed. For this reason considerable care is needed in establishing and maintaining the correct dose for the individual. Manic depression can be a devastating illness for sufferers and to those close to them. The medium- to long-term adverse effects of lithium can be very severe. Liver and thyroid damage are not uncommon. Patients on lithium must have regular blood tests to monitor the levels of the drug's metabolites in their bodies. If these are allowed build up to high levels the consequences are very dangerous. Evidence suggests that patients are unlikely to get much benefit from lithium unless they remain on it for two years. Those who stop the treatment before the two years have elapsed may be at risk of more frequent periods of illness.

LITHIUM CARBONATE

Trade name	Description
Camcolit 250	250 mg white tablets marked Camcolit.
Camcolit 400	400 mg white tablets marked Camcolit S.
Liskonum	450 mg white tablets.
Priadel	200 mg white tablets marked P200.
	400 mg white tablets marked PRIADEL.

LITHIUM CITRATE

Trade name	Description
Litarex	564 mg white tablets.

General information

Lithium is used to stabilise the moods of people suffering from manic depression and to prevent both the depressive lows and manic peaks. It is not a cure for the illness, but it does help many sufferers to lead productive and enjoyable lives by stabilising their moods. Lithium does not work for all patients, neither does it affect all patients uniformly. Whilst taking lithium care must be taken to ensure an adequate fluid and salt intake. Patients should drink at least four to six pints of liquid a day, but use alcohol in moderation because it can cause bodily fluid loss. It is also wise to take at least an average amount of salt with food. Hot weather and heavy work which causes sweating can be hazardous when on lithium. At the outset of treatment it is necessary to have the efficiency of kidneys and thyroid glands checked. Before maintenance treatment is begun the dose level for the particular patient has to be established. This is done by testing the serum level (the concentration of lithium in the blood) of lithium on the fourth and seventh days of treatment, and thereafter every seven days until the appropriate dose level has been established and stabilised. It may take a number of attempts before the correct dose for an individual patient is established. Blood tests should be repeated monthly until the dose has been stabilised for some time, after which they may be given at slightly longer intervals. These tests are vitally important, not only to prevent damage to the patient's health from too high levels of lithium, but also to reduce the risk of a relapse should the level get too low.

Dosage information

Adult (16 and over): *Lithium carbonate:* Treatment begins with 0.25–2 g per day, adjusted to the level appropriate for the individual patient.

Lithium citrate: Treatment begins with 564 mg twice daily, adjusted to the level appropriate for the individual patient.

Elderly and physically frail: Elderly and physically frail people should receive reduced dosage.

Children: Lithium is not suitable for the treatment of children.

Side effects and further information

Early side effects are: Increased thirst. Increased urination. Nausea. Mild stomach upsets. Trembling hands. Slight muscular weakness. Dry mouth. Decreased interest in sex. Slight dizziness. Aggravated acne.

Intermediate side effects are: Excessive weight gain. Excessive urination. Skin rash. Kidney damage. Damage to the thyroid gland, causing tiredness, slowing of mental processes, dry skin, aching muscles, feelings of cold and trembling hands.

Serious side effects are: Persistent diarrhoea. Severe nausea and vomiting. Severe hand tremors. Frequent muscular twitching. Blurred vision. Confusion. Serious discomfort. Goitre (a benign swelling of the thyroid gland). These serious side effects could be caused by the level of lithium in the blood becoming dangerously high. Urgent medical attention must be sought.

Conditions in which lithium should be avoided

Kidney disease. Heart disease. Addison's disease (a condition in which there is an inadequate secretion of certain hormones in the adrenal glands, causing weakness, loss of energy, low blood pressure and darkening of the skin). Pregnancy and breast-feeding.

Conditions in which lithium should be used with caution

Treatment with diuretics (which increase urination). The long-term use of lithium causes changes in the kidneys and to the thyroid gland. Therefore it is clear that lithium should be used only for severe manic depressive psychosis. It is recommended that the use of lithium should be very carefully reviewed after three to five years, with a view to stopping it. Caution is necessary in elderly and physically frail people, when reduced doses should be used.

Use in pregnancy and breast-feeding

Women who are not pregnant at the start of treatment with lithium may be offered contraceptive advice and counselling. If a woman becomes pregnant whilst taking lithium serious consideration may be given to stopping the lithium or substituting it with another less-hazardous medication, such as an antipsychotic or an antidepressant. Lithium is hazardous to the unborn child. Very sensitive judgements must be made in balancing the needs of the mother against those of the child.

CARBAMAZEPINE

Trade name	Description
Under generic name	100 mg white tablets.
	200 mg white tablets.
	400 mg white tablets.
Tegretol	100 mg white tablets marked TEGRETOL 100.
	200 mg white tablets marked TEGRETOL 200.
	400 mg white tablets marked GEIGY/GEIGY on one side TEGRETOL on the other.

General information

Carbamazepine is most often used as a treatment for epilepsy but it is also sometimes used in the treatment of manic depression and mood swings for patients who do not have a good response to lithium.

Dosage information

Treatment begins with 400 mg per day in divided doses which may be increased if necessary until the desired effect is achieved to **a maximum dose of 1600 mg per day**. Usual dose is between 400–600 mg/per day.

Elderly and physically frail: Treatment begins with a lower starting dose and should be increased in smaller steps than for healthy adults.

Children: Treatment should begin at a low dose increasing to a dose based on the formula of 10–20 mg per kilo of body weight. The manufacturers recommend that blood tests are used to monitor serum levels of the drug.

Side effects and further information

The side effects of carbamazepine are less likely to be distressing if the treatment is started by gradually increasing the dose until the desired effect of stabilising the mood swings in manic depression have been achieved. They are also said to become less of a problem to the patient after about two weeks of treatment. A wide range of side effects have been reported in patients using carbamazepine but not all patients will experience all of these: Dizziness. Headache. Visual disturbances. In elderly patients confusion and agitation. Dry mouth. Nausea. Diarrhoea. Loss of appetite. Tiredness. Ataxia (unsteady walk, shaky movements and difficulty with speech). Skin rashes (possibly three in every

PART FIVE

Central Nervous System Stimulants

Introduction

Central nervous system (CNS) stimulants are drugs which can cause feelings of excitement, tension, increased energy, euphoria and paranoia. The best-known CNS stimulants are amphetamines which are probably most well known for their reputation as recreational drugs and are often collectively referred to as 'uppers' or 'speed'. Amphetamines and similar drugs can cause dependence very rapidly and once hooked, regular users need to increase the doses they take in order to ward off the profound depression that comes when the level of the drug in their bodies falls. Nowadays CNS stimulants have very few uses in medicine. They have been used to treat depression, but this was abandoned when experience showed that not only were they ineffective, they often made people feel worse and gave them a drug problem in the process. Stimulants have also been promoted and prescribed as 'anorexiants' or appetite suppressants and the use of these drugs as slimming aids has led to many women becoming hooked on them, only to find themselves and their drug problems abandoned when CNS stimulants went out of fashion with the doctors who had previously prescribed them so freely.

CNS stimulants are now suggested for three purposes: to treat narcolepsy, to lift the moods of people suffering from 'institutionalism' or recovering from illness, and to make so-called 'hyperkinetic' (overactive) children more obedient and attentive. Narcolepsy is a very rare condition where sufferers have a powerful tendency to fall asleep in quiet surroundings or whilst engaged in monotonous activities. Institutionalism is a state of mind and is caused by long periods of living in depersonalising institutions,

100 patients). Regular blood tests are recommended as carbamazepine sometimes causes serious blood disorders.

Conditions in which carbamazepine should be avoided
People taking MAOI antidepressants. Atrioventricular abnormalities (muscles in the heart which control rate of heart beat).

Conditions in which carbamazepine should be used with caution
Severe heart disease. Kidney disease. Liver disease.

of which the most extreme examples are mental hospitals and prisons. The individual adapts to the rhythms and demands of the institution to the extent that his or her capacity to act independently or cope outside the institution is seriously impaired. Often the institutionalised individual becomes apathetic, dependent on others and lacks any sense of cause and effect in his or her own behaviour. The problems of institutionalism can be all the more severe in mental hospitals, where patients spend years on end permanently and routinely sedated by powerful drugs. Mental hospital staff often refer to their institutionalised patients as 'burnt-out schizophrenics', thus conveniently attributing their condition to the disease rather than to the institution. The victims of institutionalism can still be seen in the wards of mental hospitals twitching their nicotine-stained fingers as they watch children's television. They can also be seen in day centres performing mindless tasks euphemistically described as occupational or industrial 'therapy'. The manufacturers of Villescon, a compound combining a mild stimulant with vitamins, include 'institutional neuroses' amongst the recommended uses for their product.

All the stimulants listed in the British National Formulary are suggested as being potentially useful for the treatment of hyperkinesis in children. Whilst it is by no means controversial that some children are overactive, the medical labels given to this age-old and universal problem are very controversial indeed. Youngsters who might otherwise be described as bloody little nuisances are be transformed into medical problems by attaching impressive labels to their behaviour. Thus, Denis the Menace, Beryl the Peril and Just William might, if they lived in the real world, be diagnosed as suffering from the 'Hyperkinetic Syndrome', 'Minimal Brain Dysfunction', 'Functional Behaviour Problems' or 'Hyperkinetic Impulse Disorder', and be prescribed drugs to treat their psychiatric problems. These 'diagnoses' are very broadly defined. Overactivity, short attention span, poor powers of concentration, low frustration tolerance, impulsive and explosive temperament – these have become 'symptoms' of these childhood 'disorders'. Once the diagnosis has been made Denis, Beryl and William will be given a prescribed quantity of speed (whoops! I mean methylphenidate hydrochloride) and they will be stoned – I mean cured. This stimulant, we are told, has a paradoxical effect on hyperkintic youth. Might a similar effect might be achieved with a snort of cocaine or a tab of ecstasy?

Drugs such as amphetamines retard children's growth and there is a lack of evidence as to whether this retarded growth is made up later in the child's life or whether it is permanent. Long-term cohort studies of children treated with stimulants do not show that their prospects in adult life are enhanced by the treatment. The pharmaceutical industry has played a major part in promoting the diagnosis of hyperactivity syndrome. In the United States the pharmaceutical giant CIBA actively encouraged its salesmen to promote their product, Ritalin FBP (Functional Behaviour Problems), amongst teachers, social workers and probation officers and this early promotional activity was extremely influential. In 1973, Grinspoon and Singer, two workers at Harvard University, concluded in a scholarly review of the use of amphetamines amongst children in America that 'the possible adverse effects of these drugs and their unknown long-term risks require that we reconsider the present policy of amphetamines in the schools'.[1] Three years before they conducted their review, a spokesman for the Food and Drugs Administration was quoted as estimating that between 150,000 and 200,000 children were being treated with these drugs in America. At the same time, the National Institute of Mental Health was suggesting that there were up to four million children 'who could benefit from these drugs'. Amphetamine use never reached anything like this scale in Britain, but the issues raised by Grinspoon and Singer have still not been resolved and are still just as important, whether they apply to hundreds of children, or hundreds of thousands.

DEXAMPHETAMINE SULPHATE

Trade name	Description
Dexedrine	5 mg white tablets marked SK&F.

General information

Dexamphetamine is a potent stimulant which is used in the treatment of narcolepsy and for the so-called hyperkinetic syndrome in children. It is the most powerful CNS stimulant in current use

[1] Grinspoon, L. and Singer, S. B.: 'Amphetamines in the Treatment of Hyperkinetic Children': *Harvard Educational Review*, 43, pp. 515–55, 1973.

in the Health Service. Dexamphetamine is a widely abused drug because of its ability to produce feelings of energetic well-being, alertness and sociability. Tolerance to these effects develops very quickly, usually within two to three weeks, which leads abusers to increase steadily the dose they take in order to ward off the feelings of agitated anxiety and profound depression which occur as the effects of the drug wear off. The high doses taken by habitual abusers often cause 'amphetamine psychosis' in which the user is tormented by paranoid fears and anxieties, delusions and hallucinations. An individual in this state is terrified by a fixed belief that he or she is being persecuted or punished, hears taunting voices, feels that insects are crawling under his or her skin, gnashes his or her teeth uncontrollably, and feels unremitting terror and rage. This state can be sufficiently severe to require admission to hospital. Not all people who use amphetamines recreationally necessarily reach this state; some users take the drug occasionally to enhance their social lives or their capacity to work. In such circumstances the greatest risk run by people who use amphetamines unlawfully is the risk of arrest and prosecution by the police.

Dosage information

For the treatment of narcolepsy. 10 mg per day in divided doses, increased if necessary to **a maximum dose of 60 mg per day**.

Children: for the treatment of hyperactive children aged between three and five: 2.5 mg daily in the morning, increased if necessary by 2.5 mg per day at weekly intervals, to **a maximum dose of 20 mg per day**.

For hyperactive children aged between six and twelve: 5–10 mg per day in the morning, increased if necessary by 5 mg per day at weekly intervals, to **a maximum dose of 40 mg per day**.

This controversial treatment should only be given in circumstances where the social and psychological needs of the child and the family can be met in an effective and sensitive manner. In many parts of the country such services are either unavailable or inadequate, and in these circumstances there is no justification for using this method of dealing with the child's problems. The long-term outcome of this treatment is uncertain. There is an unmeasured risk that the child's physical growth may be permanently impaired. There is also the risk that the child may come to believe that drugs provide an easy solution to life's problems.

Side effects and further information

There is a high risk of addiction to dexamphetamine. Whilst children are taking this drug their growth is impaired and it is not known whether or not this is a permanent effect. In the short term a marked improvement in a child's behaviour may be observed, but this may be bought at an unjustifiable risk to the child. The side effects of dexamphetamine are: Risk of tolerance leading to dependence. Agitation, restlessness and insomnia. Headaches. Dizziness. Loss of appetite. Dry mouth. Diarrhoea or constipation. Difficulty with urination. In children, tearfulness, loss of appetite and loss of weight.

Conditions in which dexamphetamine must be avoided

Heart disease. Glaucoma (a condition in which there is abnormally high pressure in the eye). Extrapyramidal disorders (disorders of those parts of the central nervous system which control certain muscular actions). Overexcited states. Hyperthyroidism (a condition in which excessive amounts of thyroid hormones in the bloodstream cause rapid heart beat, tremors, anxiety, sweating, increased appetite, loss of weight and intolerance of heat). Where there is a history of drug dependency.

Conditions in which dexamphetamine should be used with caution

Insomnia. Caution is advised when used with antidepressants, anaesthetics, remedies for coughs and colds and treatments for high blood pressure.

PEMOLINE

Trade name	Description
Volital	20 mg white tablets marked P9.

General information

Pemoline is described as a weak CNS (central nervous system) stimulant and is suggested for the treatment of hyperactivity in children under specialist psychiatric supervision.

Dosage information

Children: Under the age of 6 years not recommended. For children over the age of six, treatment begins with 20 mg in the morning increasing by weekly increases of 20 mg to 60 mg each morning, increased if necessary to **a maximum dose of 120 mg each morning**.

Side effects and further information
Pemoline has been described as having a stimulant effect somewhere between caffeine and amphetamines. It has a mild alerting effect and may give a feeling of well-being. Side effects are said to be infrequent and mild, but it would be unwise and unhelpful for it to be taken too close to bedtime as it is likely to cause insomnia, its most common side effect. Other side effects which may be experienced are rapid heart beat, agitation and weight loss. Long-term use may retard growth in children.

Conditions in which pemoline should be avoided
Glaucoma (a condition in which there is abnormally high pressure in the eye). Extrapyramidal disorders (disorders of those parts of the central nervous system which control certain muscular actions). Overexcited states. Hyperthyroidism (a condition in which excessive amounts of thyroid hormones in the bloodstream cause rapid heart beat, tremors, anxiety, sweating, increased appetite, loss of weight and intolerance of heat).

Conditions in which pemoline should be used with caution
Insomnia. Caution is advised when used with antidepressants, anaesthetics, remedies for coughs and colds and treatments for high blood pressure.

PART SIX

Resources

Getting the most out of your doctor

When you are prescribed a psychiatric drug it is important that you understand what the drug is, how you should take it and what effects it will have on you. You may wish to know whether there are any alternative treatments to the proposed drug. You may want to ask whether psychotherapy or some other form of psychological treatment is available, either as an alternative to the drug, or whether psychological help might help you to recover sooner. When you know all the facts and have considered your options you may decide against taking the drug. Depending on the seriousness of your mental health problem and your circumstances, it may be unwise for you not to take the medication. All decisions on treatment involve balancing its benefits against its unwanted effects. The following list of questions for your doctor should help you to make your decision and to get the most out of your treatment.

1. **What and how?**
   - What kind of medicine is it?
   - How can it help me?
   - How and when should I take it?
   - What should I do if I miss a dose?
   - How will I know that it works?

2. **How important is it?**
   - How important is it that I take it?
   - What may happen if I do not take it?
   - What should I do if I miss a dose?

3. What side effects?
- Does it have any side effects?
- How likely is it that I will experience these side effects?
- Does taking it for a long time have any risks or dangers?
- Can I drive whilst taking it?
- Can I drink alcohol whilst taking it?
- Is it safe to take other medicines whilst taking it?
- Are there any foods I should avoid whilst taking it?

4. How long?
- How long should I continue taking it?
- When will I need to see you again?
- What will you need to know when I see you again?

If you are worried about any aspect of the treatment or uncertain about the advice you have been given and are unable to resolve these with your doctor, you may ask to be referred to another doctor for a second opinion.

Translating your prescription

When your doctor issues a prescription he may use the scholarly language of Latin to convey to the pharmacist instructions as to how and when the prescribed medication should be administered. The pharmacist then feeds these instructions into a computer which translates and prints them in modern English for you to read on a label. The following glossary of the abbreviations used by doctors to write prescriptions will help you to translate them, assuming of course, that you can read your doctor's handwriting!

a.c.	*ante cibos*	before meals
ad	*ad*	to make (a total)
ad. lib.	*ad libitum*	as much as required
b.d.		
b.i.d.	*bis in die sumendum*	twice daily
b.d.s.		
c	*cum*	with
caps.	*capsules*	
c.m.s.	*cras mane sumendum*	take tomorrow morning
c.n.	*cras nocte*	take tomorrow evening

d. } det. }	*detur*	give
e.m.p.	*ex modo prescripto*	as directed
f. } ft. }	*fiat*	make up
Gtt.	*guttae*	drops
g. or G, Gm	*grammum*	gram
haust.	*haustus*	draught
h.n.	*hac nocte*	tonight
hor. decub.	*hora decubitus*	at bedtime
h.s.	*hora somnii*	at bedtime
liq.	*liquor*	solution
m.et n.	*mane et nocte*	morning and evening
mane	*mane*	in the morning
m.d. } m.d.u. }	*more docto utendum*	take as directed
mg. or mgm.	*milligrammum*	milligram(s)
mist.	*mistura*	mixture
ml.		millilitre(s)
mor. sol.	*more solito*	as usual
nocte	*nocte*	at bedtime
noct. maneq.	*nocte maneque*	night and morning
n.r. } non rep. }	*non repetatur*	do not repeat
o.m.	*omni mane*	each morning
o.n.	*omni nocte*	each night
p.c.	*post cibos*	after meals
p.p.a.	*phialla prius agitata*	shake the bottle
p.r.n.	*pro re nata*	when required
pulv.	*pulvis*	powder
q.h.	*quaque hora*	every hour
q.4.h.	*quaque 4 hora*	every 4 hours
q.d.	*quater in die sumendum*	4 times a day
q.s.	*quantum sufficiat*	as much as required
rep.	*repetatur*	repeat
s.o.s.	*si opus sit*	when required
stat.	*statim*	at once
syr.	*syrupus*	syrup
tabs.	*tabellae*	tablets

t.d.		
t.d.s.	*ter in die sumendem*	three times daily
t.i.d.		
ung.	*unguentum*	ointment
ut dict.	*ut dictum*	as directed

Mental health treatment and the law

Informed consent in psychiatric treatment

In Britain the legal position on informed consent to treatment is not very clear. There is a legal requirement that consent to treatment should be based on the patient being informed as to the nature of the treatment, its purposes and any hazards associated with it. This does not mean, however, that the doctor must tell the patient about every conceivable risk attached to the treatment. He or she is only obliged to inform the patient of such risks in broad terms, and the law allows the doctor to exercise professional judgement as to what the patient is told. A doctor may not obtain valid consent by deceiving a patient about the nature or effects of a treatment. Neither may he or she exercise force or duress to obtain such consent. In an emergency a treatment may be given if it is necessary to save a life. For example, a doctor may give treatment to an unconscious patient if in the doctor's judgement that treatment is necessary to save the patient's life, or to a seriously mentally ill person who is incapable of giving a valid consent.

The legal position of patients receiving treatment for a mental illness is more complicated than that of people being treated for other illnesses. A number of factors need to be taken into account. These are:

The severity of the symptoms: The symptoms of serious mental illness can be very distressing to the patient and those around him or her. The distress felt by the patient must be the first consideration, with that of relatives or other carers second. This is not to say that the distress of relatives or other carers is unimportant, rather, that those involved in giving treatment must be clear as to whose distress or anxieties are being dealt with. It is not acceptable to pressure a patient into taking a drug or a higher dose of a drug simply for the convenience of others. The distress experienced by the patient as a result of a drug's effects or side effects may far exceed any embarrassment or inconvenience caused to others.

The strain imposed on those who care for the patient: Serious mental illness can cause people to behave in disturbed, disruptive and occasionally dangerous ways. It may be necessary to protect families from intolerable strains imposed by such behaviour in order to protect that patient's place within the family.

The risk of leaving dangerous symptoms untreated: In some instances it is necessary to give treatment in order to safeguard the safety of the patient, as well as other people.

The benefits of the treatment versus the disadvantages: As will be seen in this guide, the drugs used in psychiatry are not effective for all patients, and some of the drugs expose patients to risks without any realistic expectations of benefits being gained. For some patients the treatment may be worse than the illness, whilst for others the risks and side effects of the drugs may be a small price to pay for the relief they bring from tormenting or dangerous symptoms. The strategy of steadily increasing the doses of antipsychotic drugs when they have been shown to be ineffective is dangerous and unacceptable. There are situations in which physical restraint is more acceptable than attempts to stun people with powerful drugs.

Consent and the law

Only a very small proportion of people receiving treatment for mental illness are detained under the compulsory sections of the 1983 Mental Health Act. The minority who are liable to be detained may in certain circumstances be administered treatment without their consent. The position of patients subject to compulsory detention is set out later in this section.

All patients who are not subject to detention in hospital under the provisions of the Mental Health Act can refuse any treatment which they would rather not have. They have the same rights as anyone else to give or withhold legally valid consent, and in theory they should give such consent before they are given any treatment. In practice, however, few are either asked for consent or informed of their rights. What usually happens is that their prescription or injection is given as a matter of routine. In hospitals the medication trolley is often wheeled into the ward and patients are expected to queue passively and accept their treatment. In psychiatry, if the law on consent to treatment was observed to the letter, considerable inconvenience would be caused to those who prescribe and administer treatments. If it was observed, however, it might in time do much to improve both the quality of treatment received and the quality of relationships between patients and staff, which might ultimately lead to patients complying with treatment more readily. The main components of informed consent are as follows:

Information: The patient must be given information on the nature and purpose of the treatment and any serious side effects or hazards (the doctor is not obliged to inform the patient of *every* possible side effect or hazard but must not deceive the patient. In the current state of law the doctor is allowed to exercise professional judgement as to how much information is actually given to the patient).

Competency: The patient must be able to understand the nature and purpose of the treatment. The fact that someone is suffering from a mental disorder does not automatically mean that he is incapable of understanding the issues involved, but obviously some people will be better able to understand than others. A young person over the age of 16 has the same rights in consent procedures as an adult. The position of young people below the age of 16 is unclear, but learned opinion is that under current law children should be assumed to have the same rights as adults, unless it is clearly demonstrated that such a young person lacks the capacity to understand the issues involved. Factors which must be taken into account in these circumstances include the child's chronological age, his or her mental age and abilities, his or her mental condition and his or her capacity to make realistic and informed choices between the available alternatives.

Voluntariness: The patient must give consent without undue force, persuasion or influence being brought to bear. A consent obtained by fraud, deceit or threat is not legally valid and any person found administering treatment under such circumstances would be acting unlawfully.

The only circumstances in which a person not subject to detention under the Mental Health Act can be treated without a consent first being obtained are in circumstances of *urgent necessity*. For example, it would be lawful in an emergency to give drugs to a person suffering from mental illness in order to prevent that person from harming himself or other people. However such treatment can only be given for as long as it is necessary to bring the emergency to an end; the patient's consent must be obtained to continue treatment beyond that point.

Patients subject to detention under the provisions of the Mental Health Act 1983

People who are detained in hospitals under sections of the Mental Health Act for 72 hours or less, or remanded to hospital for a medical report, who are under guardianship or who are conditionally discharged from hospital, have the same right to refuse treatment as any other person. All other patients subject to detention in hospital may be given treatment without consent under the terms set out in Part IV of the Mental Health Act. Patients who are uncertain about their legal standing under the Act should seek clarification from the hospital staff.

Section 58 of the Mental Health Act is specifically concerned with drug treatments. Under this section patients subject to detention – with the exceptions mentioned above – can be given drugs *without* their consent for up to three months from the start of treatment. After three months, the treatment *cannot* continue unless: a) the patient gives a legally valid consent, or b) a doctor appointed by the Mental Health Act Commission (a special body set up to protect the rights of detained patients) certifies that the treatment is necessary.

Cases of urgent necessity

In cases of urgent necessity it is lawful to treat a mentally disordered person without that person's consent. In such cases the safeguards contained in Section 58 of the Mental Health Act and outlined do not apply. Section 62 of the Act sets out the terms of such urgent necessities as treatment which:

a) is immediately necessary to save the patient's life;

b) (not being irreversible) is immediately necessary to prevent a serious deterioration of his or her condition;

c) (not being irreversible or hazardous) is immediately necessary to alleviate serious suffering by the patient;

d) (not being irreversible or hazardous) is immediately necessary and represents the minimum interference necessary to prevent the patient from behaving violently or being a danger to himself or to others. The terms 'irreversible and hazardous' are explained as follows:

Treatment is irreversible if it has unfavourable irreversible physical or psychological consequences and hazardous if it entails significant physical hazard.

The legal issues surrounding consent to treatment are extremely complex and patients or relatives who need advice can contact MIND's Legal and Welfare Rights Service at the address provided on p. 162).

When things go wrong

Making a complaint

Since the first edition of this guide was written the complaints procedures connected with medical treatment have been considerably simplified and improved. The most significant of these changes is that the remit of the Health Service Commissioner (Ombudsman) has been extended to cover clinical judgement. This is a major change which MIND advocated twenty years ago in its evidence to a Parliamentary Select Committee. If you need to make a complaint about any treatment you have received you may find the following tips helpful.

Make it simple: Complaints about medical treatment are seldom simple or straightforward and it is therefore essential to clarify and simplify them as much as possible. It may be that you feel badly treated by a number of people who were at some stage directly or indirectly involved in your treatment, but remember that it is easier, and more effective, to shoot one arrow at a time. To put your complaint about one psychiatrist within a diatribe against the state of world psychiatry will not help you to get satisfaction.

Make it soon: The longer you leave it before you make your complaint the more difficult it will be to establish the facts. Institutions often have very short memories when things have gone wrong.

Get help: Get the help, advice and support of someone who is used to dealing with complaints procedures. Listen to his or her advice very carefully, and remember that although you have more knowledge of the people you are complaining about your adviser will probably know more about the people you are complaining to. Every procedure has its ground rules and traditions and your adviser will be able to help you negotiate these, and hopefully use them to your advantage.

Put it in writing and keep a copy: You need to be sure that your complaint does not get 'lost in the post', so put it in writing, date it and keep a copy. Keep copies of any correspondence or documents concerning your complaint in a file, and don't use that file as a beer mat – sometimes the appearance of a complaint may tilt the balance as to how the complaint is eventually dealt with.

Keep it brief: You may well feel moved to write a 50 page letter but it is unlikely that anyone will feel moved to read it. The longer your letter, the more likely you are to be written off as a 'nutcase'.

Don't overstate your case: Remember the value of understatement. The language you use in your complaint will create that vital first impression of what sort of person you are in the minds of those who are going to judge the merits of your complaint. Remember also that there are more cock-ups than conspiracies in life and more incompetents than conspirators in psychiatry.

Don't be bought off or bullied: If your complaint was serious, withdrawing it before it has been resolved may expose others to the same bad treatment of which you are complaining. However, it is sometimes graceful to accept a sincere apology.

Complaints procedures

Clinical judgement

Clinical judgement means a doctor exercising his or her professional judgement as to the most appropriate treatment or method of treatment for the individual in the circumstances which prevail at the time. In making such judgements doctors are guided by professional ethics, as set out in the Hippocratic Oath and other conventions, their knowledge of the patient's illness and circumstances, their training and knowledge of the treatments and services available to meet the patient's medical needs, the duties of care as set out in law, and respect for the patient's human dignity.

Making a complaint about your treatment in hospital

This procedure applies to any complaint about any aspect of the service you receive in hospital and applies in cases involving the following matters.

- The manner in which a doctor, nurse, psychologist, occupational therapist or any other professional exercises clinical or professional judgement.
- The manner in which any hospital employee deals with you or your treatment.

If you have a complaint about your treatment in a local hospital refer your complaint to the members of staff concerned. If you are dissatisfied by the way they deal with your complaint your next step is to complain to the managers of the hospital concerned. If you are dissatisfied with the way in which the hospital management deals with your complaint you proceed to the next stage and register your complaint with your Local Health Authority. The Health Authority will then set up a panel to review your complaint. If after the Local Health Authority has reviewed and ruled on your complaint you are still not satisfied you then proceed to the final stage and lodge your complaint with the Health Service Commissioner.

Complaining about your general practitioner

If you wish to make a complaint about any of the treatment you receive from your general practitioner you first complain to the practice concerned. If you are dissatisfied with the way in which the practice deals with your complaint your next step is to take your complaint to the Local Health Authority. The Health Authority will then set up a panel to review your complaint. If after the local Health Authority has reviewed and ruled on your complaint you are still not satisfied you then proceed to the final stage and lodge your complaint with the Health Service Commissioner.

Complaining about services provided by your local health trust

This applies to services provided by Community Nurses, Community Psychiatric Nurses, Occupational Therapists and other professionals working in and from community health centres.

Your first step is to complain to the individual or service concerned. If you are not satisfied you complain to the hospital trust which provides the service. If you are dissatisfied by the way they deal with your complaint your next step is to complain to the managers of the hospital concerned. If you are dissatisfied with the way in which the hospital management deals with your complaint you proceed to the next stage and register your complaint with your Local Health Authority. The Health Authority will then set up a panel to review your complaint. If after the local Health Authority has reviewed and ruled on your complaint you are still not satisfied you then proceed to the final stage and lodge your complaint with the Health Service Commissioner:

> Health Service Commissioner for England
> 11th Floor
> Millbank Tower
> Millbank
> London SW1P 4QP

Getting help with pursuing your complaint

In every health district there is a Community Health Council (CHC) whose specific task is to represent the interests of the public to the Local Health Authority. Your local CHC will be pleased to help you in your negotiations with local health providers and to pursue any complaint you wish to make. Your local CHC is listed in your local telephone directory.

Making a complaint about the professional misconduct of a medical practitioner

Serious professional misconduct is not defined in law as it is a matter which may involve acts or omissions which are not in themselves unlawful. Thus, a doctor would be judged guilty of serious professional misconduct if he or she had a sexual relationship with a patient. Other examples of professional misconduct might be breaching a confidential relationship, carelessly or improperly prescribing drugs, and improperly issuing medical certificates. It may involve behaviour which is damaging to the reputation of the medical profession, such as indecency, dishonesty or personally abusing drugs. Complaints should be made to:

The General Medical Council,
44 Hallam Street, London W1N 6AE

Making a complaint about the professional misconduct of a registered or enrolled nurse

Complaints should be made to:

The English Board of Nursing,
Midwifery and Health Visiting,
Victory House,
170 Tottenham Court Road,
London W1P OHA

Making a complaint about compulsory admission to a mental hospital or any treatment received whilst detained in hospital

In the first instance you must make any complaints about your detention or the treatment you received as a detained patient to the managers of the hospital in which you are detained or subject to detention. If you are not satisfied by the response from the hospital managers you can write directly to:

The Mental Health Act Commission,
Maid Marian House,
56 Houndsgate,
Nottingham NG1 6BG

Useful addresses

MIND (National Association for Mental Health)
Granta House,
15/19 The Broadway,
London E15 4BR

Wales MIND,
23 St Mary Street,
Cardiff CF1 2AA

Scottish Association for Mental Health,
40 Shandwell Place,
Edinburgh, EH2 4RT

National Schizophrenia Fellowship,
78/79 Victoria Road,
Surbiton, Surrey

The Manic Depression Fellowship,
13 Rosslyn Road,
Twickenham,
Middlesex TW1 2AR

The Northern Ireland Association for Mental Health,
Beacon House,
University Street,
Belfast

Index

ALL IN THE MIND?

Think your self better

Brian Roet

Have you a problem that won't go away? This book offers a key to solving long-term problems, physical, social and emotional. Drawing on his practical experience, Dr Roet shows how the mind plays a major role in causing and maintaining illness, and how many physical and psychological symptoms are messages from the unconscious.

By unravelling our thought processes and using practical self-help techniques, Dr Roet shows everyone how they can start on the road to self-knowledge and recovery.

PERSONAL THERAPY

How to change your life for the better

Brian Roet

In this book Dr Roet shows us how therapeutic techniques can be used to release deep-seated emotions, acknowledge our strengths and weaknesses and establish emotional eqilibrium. His reassuring and practical advice guides us towards new ways to enjoy a more fulfilling life.

Case studies are used to inform and advise readers of the benefits of personal therapy and how it can play an active role in helping the mind resolve anxieties and even disease.

DEALING WITH DEPRESSION

Whatever you're going through, we'll go through it with you

Trevor Barnes with The Samaritans

This practical and inspiring guide has been written to offer support to all those in crisis and their families. It is for all who are familiar with feelings of despair, or who believe that they can no longer face the future – and for those who care about them.

Written and endorsed by The Samaritans, this important book draws on over 40 years collective experience, to provide self-help methods for befriending and listening to yourself and to others – to bring about positive and constructive change for the future.

PANIC ATTACKS

A practical guide to recognising and dealing with feelings of panic

Sue Breton

Panic attacks can ruin your life – but it lies within your power to overcome your fears. Sue Breton, clinical psychologist, researcher and former sufferer, shows you how to help yourself by recognising situations and symptoms which trigger an attack, understanding what type of attack you have and taking short term action to suit your personal needs.

The techniques and advice given in this book will give you power over panic for good.

ANXIETY AND DEPRESSION

A Practical guide to recovery

Professor Robert Priest

Feelings of anxiety and depression confront us all from time to time, and can vary in their severity. Recognising the symptoms, understanding their causes and effects, and knowing what help is available can be very reassuring, and help to overcome the condition.

Professor Priest has written this book to provide help for those feeling anxious and depressed. He covers practical self help methods of reducing stress and offers an explanation of the causes and effects of anxiety and depression. This book provides up-to-date information on the professional help available and details the action and side-effects of medication.

DIY PSYCHOTHERAPY

A Practical guide to self-analysis

Dr Martin Shepherd

Would you like to understand yourself better? Dr Shepherd draws on his long experience as a professional therapist to present this do-it-yourself approach to psychotherapy. Each chapter focuses on one aspect of human behaviour and concludes with a series of exercises designed to give you a clearer understanding of your own thoughts and responses.

Extremely practical and easy to follow, this book will enhance your enjoyment of life, and save you a fortune in therapist's fees!

ORDER FORM

To order any of the above titles direct from Vermilion (p&p free), use the form below or call our credit-card hotline on:

01279 427 203

Please send me . . . . . . .copies of **All in the Mind?** @ £8.99 each
Please send me . . . . . . .copies of **Personal Therapy** @ £8.99 each
Please send me . . . . . . .copies of **Dealing with Depression** @ £8.99 each
Please send me . . . . . . .copies of **Panic Attacks** @ £8.99 each
Please send me . . . . . . .copies of **Anxiety and Depression** @ £8.99 each
Please send me . . . . . . .copies of **DIY Psychotherapy** @ £8.99 each

Mr/Ms/Mrs/Miss/ Other

Address:

Postcode:

Signed:

How to pay
I enclose a cheque/postal order for £ . . . . .made payable to 'VERMILION'
I wish to pay by Access/Visa card (delete where appropriate)

Card No: . . . . .Expiry Date: . . . .

Post order to **Murlyn Services Ltd, Po Box 50, Harlow, Essex CM17 0DZ.**

POSTAGE AND PACKING ARE FREE. Offer open in Great Britain including Northern Ireland. Books should arrive less than 28 days after we receive your order; they are subject to availability at time of ordering. If not entirely satisfied return in the same packaging and condition as received with a covering letter within 7 days. Vermilion books are available from all good booksellers.